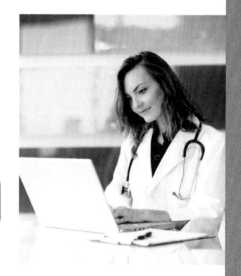

Management of High Grade Bladder Cancer: A Multidisciplinary Approach

Editors

ARJUN V. BALAR
MATTHEW I. MILOWSKY

UROLOGIC CLINICS
OF NORTH AMERICA

www.urologic.theclinics.com

Consulting Editor
SAMIR S. TANEJA

May 2015 • Volume 42 • Number 2

ELSEVIER

1600 John F. Kennedy Boulevard ● Suite 1800 ● Philadelphia, Pennsylvania, 19103-2899

http://www.theclinics.com

UROLOGIC CLINICS OF NORTH AMERICA Volume 42, Number 2
May 2015 ISSN 0094-0143, ISBN-13: 978-0-323-37623-5

Editor: Kerry Holland
Developmental Editor: Susan Showalter

Urologic Clinics of North America (ISSN 0094-0143) is published quarterly by Elsevier Inc., 360 Park Avenue South, New York, NY 10010-1710. Months of issue are February, May, August, and November. Business and Editorial Offices: 1600 John F. Kennedy Blvd., Suite 1800, Philadelphia, PA 19103-2899. Periodicals postage paid at New York, NY and additional mailing offices. Subscription prices are $355.00 per year (US individuals), $602.00 per year (US institutions), $415.00 per year (Canadian individuals), $752.00 per year (Canadian institutions), $515.00 per year (foreign individuals), and $752.00 per year (foreign institutions). Foreign air speed delivery is included in all *Clinics* subscription prices. All prices are subject to change without notice. **POSTMASTER:** Send address changes to *Urologic Clinics of North America*, Elsevier Health Sciences Division, Subscription Customer Service, 3251 Riverport Lane, Maryland Heights, MO 63043. Customer Service: 1-800-654-2452 (US). From outside the United States, call 1-314-447-8871. Fax: 1-314-447-8029. E-mail: JournalsCustomerServiceusa@elsevier.com (for print support) and JournalsOnlineSupport-usa@elsevier.com (for online support).

Reprints. For copies of 100 or more, of articles in this publication, please contact the Commercial Reprints Department, Elsevier Inc., 360 Park Avenue South, New York, New York 10010-1710. Tel.: 212-633-3874; Fax: 212-633-3820; E-mail: reprints@elsevier.com.

Urologic Clinics of North America is covered in MEDLINE/PubMed (*Index Medicus*), *Excerpta Medica, Current Contents/Clinical Medicine, Science Citation Index,* and *ISI/BIOMED*.

PROGRAM OBJECTIVE
The goal of *Urologic Clinics of North America* is to keep practicing urologists and urology residents up to date with current clinical practice in urology by providing timely articles reviewing the state of the art in patient care.

TARGET AUDIENCE
Practicing urologists, urology residents and other health care professionals practicing in the discipline of urology.

LEARNING OBJECTIVES
Upon completion of this activity, participants will be able to:
1. Review different surgical approaches to the treatment of bladder cancer.
2. Discuss the use of drug therapies in the management of localized bladder cancer.
3. Recognize new and developing methods of bladder cancer treatment.

ACCREDITATION
The Elsevier Office of Continuing Medical Education (EOCME) is accredited by the Accreditation Council for Continuing Medical Education (ACCME) to provide continuing medical education for physicians.

The EOCME designates this enduring material for a maximum of 15 *AMA PRA Category 1 Credit*(s)™. Physicians should claim only the credit commensurate with the extent of their participation in the activity.

All other health care professionals requesting continuing education credit for this enduring material will be issued a certificate of participation.

DISCLOSURE OF CONFLICTS OF INTEREST
The EOCME assesses conflict of interest with its instructors, faculty, planners, and other individuals who are in a position to control the content of CME activities. All relevant conflicts of interest that are identified are thoroughly vetted by EOCME for fair balance, scientific objectivity, and patient care recommendations. EOCME is committed to providing its learners with CME activities that promote improvements or quality in healthcare and not a specific proprietary business or a commercial interest.

The planning committee, staff, authors and editors listed below have identified no financial relationships or relationships to products or devices they or their spouse/life partner have with commercial interest related to the content of this CME activity:
Piyush K. Agarwal, MD; Emanuela Altobelli, MD; Andrea B. Apolo, MD; Arjun Balar, MD; Bernard H. Bochner, MD; Brock E. Boehm, DO; Eugene K. Cha, MD; Deborah E. Citrin, MD; Michela de Martino, PhD; Timothy F. Donahue, MD; Anjali Fortna; Peter Greene, MD; Kerry Holland; Gopa Iyer, MD; David C. Johnson, MD, MPH; Emmet Jordan, MB BCh, BAO, MRCPI; Tobias Klatte, MD; Joseph C. Liao, MD; Indu Kumari; Matthew I. Milowsky, MD; Anirban P. Mitra, MD, PhD; Christopher Premo, MD; John P. Sfakianos, MD; Megan Suermann; Robert S. Svatek, MD, MSCI; Dimitar V. Zlatev, MD.

The planning committee, staff, authors and editors listed below have identified financial relationships or relationships to products or devices they or their spouse/life partner have with commercial interest related to the content of this CME activity:
Matthew D. Galsky, MD is a consultant/advisor for Merck & Co., Inc; Astellas Pharma US, Inc; and BioMotiv; has research support from Bristol-Myers Squibb Company; and stock ownership in Dual Therapeutics, a BioMotiv company.
Seth P. Lerner, MD, FACS is a consultant/advisor for Biocancell; Vaxxion Therapeutics; Genentech, A member of the Roche Group; Merck & Co., Inc; Sitka Biopharma; Neuclexx; TheraCoat; and has research support from Endo Pharmaceuticals Inc; and FKD Therapies Oy.
Ilaria Lucca, MD has research grants from the The European Urological Scholarship Programme and the Development Fund of the University Hospital of Lausanne, Switzerland.
Matthew E. Nielsen, MD, MS is a consultant/advisor for Grand Rounds and the American College of Physicians.
Shahrokh F. Shariat, MD is on the speakers bureau for Ely Lilly and Company; Astellas Pharma US, Inc; Takeda Pharmaceutical Company Limited; Janssen Pharmaceuticals, Inc.; Ipsen Biopharmaceuticals, Inc; and Olympus Corporation; is a consultant/advisor for Astellas Pharma US, Inc; Ipsen Biopharmaceuticals, Inc; Wolff; and Olympus Corporation.
Samir S. Taneja, MD is a consultant/advisor for Bayer HealthCare AG; Eigen Pharma LLC; GTx, Inc.; HealthTronics, Inc.; and Hitachi, Ltd.

UNAPPROVED/OFF-LABEL USE DISCLOSURE
The EOCME requires CME faculty to disclose to the participants:
1. When products or procedures being discussed are off-label, unlabelled, experimental, and/or investigational (not US Food and Drug Administration [FDA] approved); and
2. Any limitations on the information presented, such as data that are preliminary or that represent ongoing research, interim analyses, and/or unsupported opinions. Faculty may discuss information about pharmaceutical agents that is outside of FDA-approved labelling. This information is intended solely for CME and is not intended to promote off-label use of these

medications. If you have any questions, contact the medical affairs department of the manufacturer for the most recent prescribing information.

TO ENROLL
To enroll in the *Urologic Clinics of North America* Continuing Medical Education program, call customer service at 1-800-654-2452 or sign up online at http://www.theclinics.com/home/cme. The CME program is available to subscribers for an additional annual fee of USD $270.

METHOD OF PARTICIPATION
In order to claim credit, participants must complete the following:
1. Complete enrolment as indicated above.
2. Read the activity.
3. Complete the CME Test and Evaluation. Participants must achieve a score of 70% on the test. All CME Tests and Evaluations must be completed online.

CME INQUIRIES/SPECIAL NEEDS
For all CME inquiries or special needs, please contact elsevierCME@elsevier.com.

Contributors

CONSULTING EDITOR

SAMIR S. TANEJA, MD
The James M. Neissa and Janet Riha Neissa
Professor of Urologic Oncology; Professor of
Urology and Radiology; Director, Division of
Urologic Oncology; Co-Director, Smilow
Comprehensive Prostate Cancer Center,
Department of Urology, NYU Langone Medical
Center, New York, New York

EDITORS

ARJUN V. BALAR, MD
Assistant Professor of Medicine; Co-Leader,
Genitourinary Cancers Program, Laura and
Isaac Perlmutter Cancer Center at NYU
Langone, New York, New York

MATTHEW I. MILOWSKY, MD
Associate Professor of Medicine; Section
Chief, Genitourinary Oncology; Co-Director,
Urologic Oncology Program, UNC Lineberger
Comprehensive Cancer Center, Chapel Hill,
North Carolina

AUTHORS

PIYUSH K. AGARWAL, MD
Head, Bladder Cancer Section, Urologic
Oncology Branch, National Cancer Institute,
National Institutes of Health, Bethesda,
Maryland

EMANUELA ALTOBELLI, MD
Department of Urology, Stanford University
School of Medicine, Stanford, California;
Department of Urology, Campus Biomedico
University, Rome, Italy

ANDREA B. APOLO, MD
Chief, Bladder Cancer Section, Genitourinary
Malignancies Branch, Center for Cancer
Research, National Cancer Institute,
National Institutes of Health, Bethesda,
Maryland

ARJUN V. BALAR, MD
Assistant Professor of Medicine; Co-Leader,
Genitourinary Cancers Program, Laura and
Isaac Perlmutter Cancer Center at NYU
Langone, New York, New York

BERNARD H. BOCHNER, MD
Attending, Urology Service, Department of
Surgery, Memorial Sloan Kettering Cancer
Center, New York, New York

BROCK E. BOEHM, DO
Adult Cancer Program, Department of Urology,
Cancer Therapy and Research Center, The
University of Texas Health Science Center San
Antonio, San Antonio, Texas

EUGENE K. CHA, MD
Fellow in Urologic Oncology, Urology Service,
Department of Surgery, Memorial Sloan
Kettering Cancer Center, New York, New York

DEBORAH E. CITRIN, MD
Investigator, Radiation Oncology Branch,
Center for Cancer Research, National Cancer
Institute, Bethesda, Maryland

MICHELA DE MARTINO, PhD
Department of Urology, Comprehensive
Cancer Center, Vienna General Hospital,
Medical University of Vienna, Vienna, Austria

TIMOTHY F. DONAHUE, MD
Assistant Professor of Surgery, Center for
Prostate Disease Research, Uniformed
Services University, Rockville, Maryland; John
P. Murthy Cancer Center, Urology Service,
Walter Reed National Military Medical Center,
Bethesda, Maryland

MATTHEW D. GALSKY, MD
Director of Genitourinary Medical Oncology;
Associate Professor of Medicine, The Tisch
Cancer Institute, Mount Sinai School of
Medicine, New York, New York

PETER S. GREENE, MD
Urology Resident, Department of Urology,
University of North Carolina, School of
Medicine, Chapel Hill, North Carolina

GOPA IYER, MD
Department of Medicine, Memorial Sloan
Kettering Cancer Center, New York, New York

DAVID C. JOHNSON, MD, MPH
Urology Resident, Department of Urology,
University of North Carolina, School of
Medicine, Chapel Hill, North Carolina

EMMET J. JORDAN, MB BCh, BAO, MRCPI
Department of Medicine, Memorial Sloan
Kettering Cancer Center, New York,
New York

TOBIAS KLATTE, MD
Department of Urology, Comprehensive
Cancer Center, Vienna General Hospital,
Medical University of Vienna, Vienna, Austria

SETH P. LERNER, MD, FACS
Translational Biology and Molecular Medicine
Program, Beth and Dave Swalm Chair in
Urologic Oncology; Professor of Urology, Scott
Department of Urology, Dan L. Duncan Cancer
Center, Baylor College of Medicine Medical
Center, Houston, Texas

JOSEPH C. LIAO, MD
Department of Urology, Stanford University
School of Medicine, Stanford, California;
Veterans Affairs Palo Alto Health Care System,
Palo Alto, California

ILARIA LUCCA, MD
Department of Urology, Comprehensive
Cancer Center, Vienna General Hospital,

Medical University of Vienna, Vienna,
Austria; Department of Urology, Centre
Hospitalier Universitaire Vaudois, Lausanne,
Switzerland

MATTHEW I. MILOWSKY, MD
Associate Professor of Medicine; Section
Chief, Genitourinary Oncology; Co-Director,
Urologic Oncology Program, UNC Lineberger
Comprehensive Cancer Center, Chapel Hill,
North Carolina

ANIRBAN P. MITRA, MD, PhD
Senior Research Associate, Department of
Pathology and Center for Personalized
Medicine, University of Southern California,
Los Angeles, California

MATTHEW E. NIELSEN, MD, MS
Assistant Professor of Urology, Department of
Urology, University of North Carolina, School of
Medicine, Chapel Hill, North Carolina

CHRISTOPHER PREMO, MD
Resident, Radiation Oncology Branch, Center
for Cancer Research, National Cancer Institute,
Bethesda, Maryland

JOHN P. SFAKIANOS, MD
Assistant Professor, Department of Urology,
Mount Sinai School of Medicine, New York,
New York

SHAHROKH F. SHARIAT, MD
Professor and Chairman, Department of
Urology, Comprehensive Cancer Center,
Vienna General Hospital, Medical University
of Vienna, Vienna, Austria; Adjunct Professor
of Urology, Department of Urology, University
of Texas Southwestern Medical Center, Dallas,
Texas; Adjunct Professor of Urology and
Medical Oncology, Department of Urology,
Weill Cornell Medical College, New
York-Presbyterian Hospital, Cornell University,
New York, New York

ROBERT S. SVATEK, MD, MSCI
Adult Cancer Program, Department of Urology,
Cancer Therapy and Research Center, The
University of Texas Health Science Center San
Antonio, San Antonio, Texas

DIMITAR V. ZLATEV, MD
Department of Urology, Stanford University
School of Medicine, Stanford, California

Contents

Bladder cancer ranges from a low-grade variant to high-grade disease. Assessment for treatment depends on white light cystoscopy, however because of its limitations there is a need for improved visualization of flat, multifocal, high-grade, and muscle-invasive lesions. Photodynamic diagnosis and narrow-band imaging provide additional contrast enhancement of bladder tumors and have been shown to improve detection rates. Confocal laser endomicroscopy and optical coherence tomography enable real-time, high-resolution, subsurface tissue characterization with spatial resolutions similar to histology. Molecular imaging offers the potential for the combination of optical imaging technologies with cancer-specific molecular agents to improve the specificity of disease detection.

This article summarizes strategies being investigated in patients with nonmuscle invasive bladder cancer. Progress has been made toward improving the delivery method of intravesical agents. Intravesical therapy is limited by the amount of time that the agent remains in contact with the bladder. Bladder cancer is considered to be responsive to immune therapy. Thus, many novel approaches are immune-based therapies and include cancer vaccines, use of Bacillus Calmette-Guérin (BCG) subcomponents, and checkpoint inhibitors. Finally, access to bladder mucosa via direct catheterization into the bladder via the urethra has enabled unique strategies for delivery of cancer therapy including viral- or plasmid-based gene therapy.

Radical cystectomy is a standard treatment of nonmetastatic, muscle-invasive bladder cancer. Treatment with trimodality therapy consisting of maximal transurethral resection of the bladder tumor followed by concurrent chemotherapy and radiation has emerged as a method to preserve the native bladder in highly motivated patients. Several factors can affect the likelihood of long-term bladder preservation after trimodality therapy and therefore should be taken into account when selecting patients. New radiation techniques such as intensity modulated radiation therapy and image-guided radiation therapy may decrease the toxicity of radiotherapy in this setting. Novel chemotherapy regimens may improve response rates and minimize toxicity.

Although cisplatin-based chemotherapy followed by radical cystectomy is the standard treatment of muscle-invasive bladder cancer, population-based studies reveal that only a small fraction of patients actually receive such treatment. A comprehensive understanding of the reasons for this gap between efficacy and effectiveness is necessary to increase the likelihood of cure of all patients with muscle-invasive bladder cancer. These reasons include systems-, provider-, and patient-level barriers that are not amenable to a single solution. Tackling each barrier will ultimately be necessary to bridge the disconnect between what is *achievable* and what is actually *achieved*.

Improvements in the accuracy of clinical staging and refinements in patient selection may allow for improved outcomes of bladder-preservation strategies for muscle-invasive bladder cancer incorporating radical transurethral resection (TUR) and partial cystectomy (PC). Retrospective studies of patients treated with radical cystectomy and pelvic lymph node dissection have reported an association between greater extent of lymphadenectomy and improved clinical outcomes. However, there is no consensus regarding the optimal extent of lymphadenectomy, as there are currently no reports from prospective, randomized trials to address this issue in regards to cancer-specific and overall survival. Future advances in the understanding of the appropriate extent of lymphadenectomy requires well-designed prospective clinical trials that directly compare varying extents of surgery with their ability to provide local and distant disease control and disease-specific survival.

The Cancer Genome Atlas project has identified and confirmed several important molecular alterations that form the basis for tumorigenesis and disease progression in muscle-invasive bladder cancer. Profiling studies also have reported on validated biomarker panels that predict prognosis and may be used to identify patients who require more aggressive therapy. This article describes the major molecular alterations in muscle-invasive urothelial carcinoma, and how several of these are being investigated as targets for novel therapeutics. It also highlights studies that identify biomarkers for platinum sensitivity, and efforts to integrate targeted therapeutics and companion theranostics for personalized treatment of muscle-invasive bladder cancer.

Since the advent of cisplatin-based combination therapy in the management of muscle-invasive and advanced bladder cancer, there has been little progress in improving outcomes for patients. Novel therapies beyond cytotoxic chemotherapy are needed. The neoadjuvant paradigm lends to acquiring ample pretreatment and posttreatment tumor tissue as a standard of care, which enables comprehensive biomarker analyses to better understand mechanisms of both response and resistance, which will aid drug development. This article discusses the evolution of neoadjuvant therapy as standard treatment and the role it may serve toward the development of novel therapies.

UROLOGIC CLINICS OF NORTH AMERICA

FORTHCOMING ISSUES

August 2015
Testicular Cancer
Daniel W. Lin, *Editor*

November 2015
Contemporary Antibiotic Management for Urologic Procedures and Infections
Sarah C. Flury and Anthony J. Schaeffer, *Editors*

February 2016
Biomarkers in Urologic Cancer
Kevin Loughlin, *Editor*

RECENT ISSUES

February 2015
Minimally Invasive Pediatric Urologic Surgery
Aseem R. Shukla, *Editor*

November 2014
Advances in Robotic-Assisted Urologic Surgery
Ashok Hemal, *Editor*

August 2014
Urodynamics
Benjamin M. Brucker and Victor W. Nitti, *Editors*

RELATED INTEREST

Hematology/Oncology Clinics of North America February 2015 (Vol. 29, No. 1)
Colorectal Cancer
Leonard B. Saltz, *Editor*

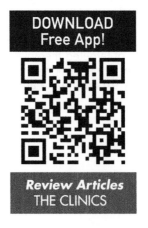

NOW AVAILABLE FOR YOUR iPhone and iPad

Foreword

Management of High Grade Bladder Cancer: A Multidisciplinary Approach

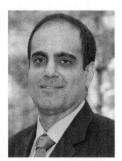

Samir S. Taneja, MD
Consulting Editor

In the battlefield of Urologic Oncology, we face two distinct enemies. First, typically on the frontline, we are confronted with low-risk variants of urologic cancers that carry high prevalence and low risk of mortality. The management of low-grade noninvasive bladder cancers, small incidental renal masses, and low-risk prostate cancers inundates our practice, but carries confusing, conflicted goals. In the case of low-risk cancers, we wish to limit detection to those cancers that are truly harmful, reduce anxiety in our patients, limit treatment while minimizing the cost of surveillance, and avoid the morbidity of unnecessary treatment. We treat the low-risk cancer most often, but, in doing so, we rarely improve longevity.

On the second line, often buried at a distant back end of the battlefield, we face our true nemesis, the lethal cancer. Most of us who do this for a living entered Urologic Oncology to save lives, but the lives that need saving are often beyond our grasp. In confronting lethal malignancies, we have learned that single-modality approaches generally fail. The use of multimodal therapy is pervasive in solid tumor oncology, but has been slow to infiltrate our own battle tactics in Urologic Oncology. Testis cancer may be the best example of success achieved through multimodal approach, and importantly, by introducing systemic therapy to

those with advanced disease, a role for surgery was carved out in the care of these patients. Now, reciprocally, systemic therapy is used efficaciously in men who would have previously been considered only for surgery. Such interactive, interdisciplinary approaches to disease serve only to elevate the game and provide better outcomes and more options for patients.

High-risk and invasive bladder cancers, as a whole, are the most lethal cancers we face in Urologic Oncology. Even with aggressive, multimodal approaches, outcomes are not nearly as good as we would like them to be. Nonetheless, our management of these lethal cancers is distinct from lethal prostate or kidney malignancies in that we have developed multimodal approaches that clearly improve survival. Furthermore, those multimodal strategies have emerged as standard of care and have created new frontiers for exploration.

In this issue of *Urologic Clinics of North America*, Drs Arjun Balar and Matthew Milowsky have put together a comprehensive series of articles outlining the multidisciplinary process that goes into optimizing care of the bladder cancer patient. The outstanding contributions of key opinion leaders in the field of bladder cancer not only illustrate the current state-of-the-art for caring for these patients but also create a strategic roadmap for where the field will go in years to come. This

Urol Clin N Am 42 (2015) xi–xii
http://dx.doi.org/10.1016/j.ucl.2015.03.002
0094-0143/15/$ – see front matter © 2015 Published by Elsevier Inc.

issue of *Urologic Clinics of North America* should not only serve to educate the reader regarding the current optimal management of invasive bladder cancer but also fuel thought regarding strategies for the development of multimodal approaches in renal and prostate malignancies as well. I would like to personally thank Drs Balar and Milowsky, and each of the contributing authors, for this wonderful issue of *Urologic Clinics of North America*.

Samir S. Taneja, MD
Division of Urologic Oncology
Smilow Comprehensive Prostate Cancer Center
Department of Urology
NYU Langone Medical Center
150 East 32nd Street, Suite 200
New York, NY 10016, USA

E-mail address:
samir.taneja@nyumc.org

Preface
Multidisciplinary Care of the Urothelial Cancer Patient

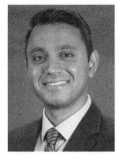 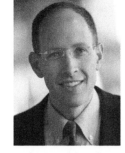

Arjun V. Balar, MD   Matthew I. Milowsky MD

Editors

Invasive urothelial cancer is a heterogeneous disease with a clear need to identify better methods to differentiate those patients who can be managed less aggressively from those who require aggressive multimodal therapy. Novel diagnostic tools, new treatments and methods for treatment delivery, modern surgical techniques, and a better understanding of the molecular underpinnings that drive the disease will assuredly improve treatment selection and lead to improved outcomes for patients.

As Guest Editors for this issue of *Urologic Clinics of North America*, we aimed to recruit thought leaders in urologic oncology, radiation oncology, and medical oncology as well as translational scientists who focus on invasive urothelial cancer to provide a comprehensive overview of the multidisciplinary care of the urothelial cancer patient. The issue begins with novel diagnostic techniques as well as new treatments and treatment delivery methods in non-muscle-invasive high-grade disease and then shifts toward the management of muscle-invasive disease with in-depth discussions focused on trimodality bladder preservation, and a thorough discussion of the conflict between the data supporting and the reality of neoadjuvant chemotherapy utilization. Also discussed is the current status of novel biomarkers to predict outcomes for localized disease after primary treatment. We next focus on the role for less aggressive surgery in muscle-invasive disease, followed by an in-depth commentary on the evolution of modern surgical techniques including robotic surgery and its clinical impact as compared with cost. The recently reported comprehensive molecular characterization of invasive urothelial cancer by The Cancer Genome Atlas project provided a new framework for the development of novel therapies, and in this issue, we also review the impact of these findings on the management of localized urothelial cancer as well as metastatic disease. We are delighted that this group of thought leaders agreed to work on this issue and we are confident that the reader will walk away with a comprehensive and up-to-date understanding of multimodal therapy in invasive urothelial cancer.

Arjun V. Balar, MD
Genitourinary Cancers Program
NYU Perlmutter Cancer Center
160 East 34th Street, 8th Floor
New York, NY 10016, USA

Matthew I. Milowsky, MD
Genitourinary Oncology
Urologic Oncology Program
UNC Lineberger Comprehensive Cancer Center
Division of Hematology/Oncology
3rd Floor, Physician's Office Building
170 Manning Drive
Chapel Hill, NC 27599, USA

E-mail addresses:
arjun.balar@nyumc.org (A.V. Balar)
matt_milowsky@med.unc.edu (M.I. Milowsky)

Urol Clin N Am 42 (2015) xiii
http://dx.doi.org/10.1016/j.ucl.2015.03.001
0094-0143/15/$ – see front matter © 2015 Published by Elsevier Inc.

Preface

Multidisciplinary Care of the Urothelial Cancer Patient

Advances in Imaging Technologies in the Evaluation of High-Grade Bladder Cancer

 CrossMark

Dimitar V. Zlatev, MD[a], Emanuela Altobelli, MD[a,b],
Joseph C. Liao, MD[a,c],*

KEYWORDS

- Bladder cancer • Confocal laser endomicroscopy • Fluorescence cystoscopy • Molecular imaging
- Narrow band imaging • Optical coherence tomography • Photodynamic diagnosis

KEY POINTS

- Improved optical imaging of the bladder can lead to more effective use of bladder-sparing management for low-grade cancer and more aggressive treatment for high-grade cancer.
- Photodynamic diagnosis and narrow band imaging are macroscopic imaging modalities and provide contrast enhancement of suspicious lesions that improve detection rates.
- Confocal laser endomicroscopy is an example of a microscopic optical biopsy technology that provides high-resolution and subsurface tissue characterization similar to histology.
- Confocal laser endomicroscopy is the only clinical technology capable of differentiating high-grade and low-grade bladder cancer.
- The highest image resolution is inferred by molecular specificity. The development of molecular markers and binding agents for molecular imaging can serve to differentiate low-grade and high-grade disease.

INTRODUCTION

Bladder cancer is the sixth most common cancer in the United States with 74,690 new cases and 15,580 deaths expected in 2014.[1] The natural history of bladder cancer is heterogeneous, ranging from low-grade variant that does not recur after local resection to a high-grade subtype that recurs and progresses to metastatic, lethal disease.[2] Although 80% of patients present at a non–muscle-invasive stage (Ta, T1, TIS) that may be managed endoscopically, recurrence rate reaches 61% at 1 year and 78% at 5 years.[3,4] As a result of its high recurrence rate and associated need for lifelong surveillance and repeat resections, the health care costs for bladder cancer are among the highest of all malignancies.[3,5]

White light cystoscopy (WLC) is the standard for evaluation of bladder urothelium. In the office setting, flexible cystoscopes are used for initial

Dr J.C. Liao is supported in part by grant National Institutes of Health (NIH) R01 CA160986.
Conflict of Interest: Dr D.V. Zlatev and Dr E. Altobelli declare no potential conflicts of interest relevant to this article. Dr J.C. Liao received research support from the NIH (R01 CA160986) and travel support from Mauna Kea Technologies, including expenses covered or reimbursed.
a Department of Urology, Stanford University School of Medicine, 300 Pasteur Drive, Room S-287, Stanford, CA 94305-5118, USA; b Department of Urology, Campus Biomedico, Via Alvaro del Portillo 200, Rome 00128, Italy; c Urology Section, Veterans Affairs Palo Alto Health Care System, 3801 Miranda Avenue, Palo Alto, CA 94304, USA
* Corresponding author. 300 Pasteur Drive, Room S-287, Stanford, CA 94305-5118.
E-mail address: jliao@stanford.edu

Urol Clin N Am 42 (2015) 147–157
http://dx.doi.org/10.1016/j.ucl.2015.01.001
0094-0143/15/$ – see front matter Published by Elsevier Inc.

identification of suspected lesions and subsequent surveillance for recurrence. In the operating room, complete transurethral resection (TUR) with larger rigid cystoscopes is performed for tissue diagnosis and local staging. Despite its central role, WLC has well-recognized limitations.[6,7] Although sufficient for the identification of papillary lesions, visual appearance under white light is unreliable for the determination of low- and high-grade cancer and cannot assess level of invasion.[8] Additionally, nonpapillary and flat malignant lesions such as carcinoma in situ (CIS) can be difficult to differentiate from inflammation,[6] with detection rates of CIS only 58% to 68% by WLC.[9–11] Smaller or satellite tumors can be missed, which contributes to the up to 40% rate of residual bladder cancer found at the time of 'second-look' TUR.[12,13] Finally, indistinct borders and difficult visualization of submucosal tumor margins during TUR can lead to incomplete tumor resection and understaging of bladder cancer.[14,15] These limitations of WLC contribute to the increased risk of cancer persistence, recurrence, and in the case of high-grade bladder cancer, progression to metastatic lethal disease.[2,16,17]

To address the shortcomings of WLC, several adjunctive optical imaging technologies have emerged with the goal to improve bladder cancer detection and resection (**Table 1**). The imaging technologies can be broadly categorized based on their field of view. Photodynamic diagnosis (PDD) and narrow band imaging (NBI) are examples of macroscopic imaging modalities that survey a large area of mucosa, similar to WLC, but provide additional contrast enhancement to distinguish suspicious lesions from noncancerous mucosa. Microscopic modalities including optical coherence tomography (OCT) and confocal laser endomicroscopy (CLE) provide high-resolution, subsurface tissue characterization similar to histology and thus offer the potential for 'optical biopsy' of bladder cancer. Molecular imaging, through coupling of optical imaging technologies with fluorescently labeled binding agents (eg, antibodies), may enable real-time cancer imaging with molecular specificity. These technological advances have the potential to improve optical diagnosis and endoscopic management of bladder cancer. The most recent literature on adjunctive optical imaging technologies is reviewed, with consideration for the evaluation of high-grade bladder cancer highlighted.

PHOTODYNAMIC DIAGNOSIS

PDD, also known as fluorescence cystoscopy or blue light cystoscopy, provides wide-field fluorescence imaging of the bladder with a field of view comparable to WLC. PDD requires preoperative intravesical administration of a photosensitive

Table 1
Characteristics and properties of adjunct optical imaging technologies for bladder cancer

Name	Mechanism	Contrast Agent	Resolution	Depth	Scope or Probe (Diameter)	Status
PDD	Fluorescence	HAL	mm – cm	Surface	Standard rigid cystoscope	Clinical
NBI	Absorption	None	mm – cm	Surface	Flexible cystoscope (5.5 mm) or standard rigid cystoscope	Clinical
CLE	Fluorescence	Fluorescein	1–3.5 μm	120 μm	Probe (0.85–2.6 mm)	Clinical/investigational (in vivo)
OCT	Scattering	None	10–20 μm	∼2.5 mm	Probe (2.7 mm)	Clinical/investigational (in vivo)
Raman	Scattering	Optional (SERS)	—	2 mm	Probe (2.1 mm)	Investigational (in vivo)
UV	Fluorescence	None	mm – cm	Surface	Probe (3 mm)	Investigational (in vivo)
SFE	Reflectance + fluorescence	None	mm – cm	Surface	Scope/Probe (1.2 mm)	Investigational (ex vivo)

Abbreviations: CLE, confocal laser endomicroscopy; HAL, hexaminolevulinate; NBI, narrow band imaging; OCT, optical coherence tomography; PDD, photodynamic diagnosis; SERS, surface-enhanced Raman scattering; SFE, scanning fiber endoscopy; UV, ultraviolet.

protoporphyrin IX precursor as the contrast agent, a blue light source that illuminates at 375 to 440 nm, and a specialized lens and camera head. Once taken up by the bladder urothelium, the protoporphyrin accumulates preferentially in neoplastic cells and emits a fluorescence in the red part of the spectrum under blue light excitation, allowing visualization of the tumor (**Fig. 1**).[18] Two protoporphyrin analogues, 5-aminolevulinic acid and its ester derivative hexaminolevulinate, have been investigated clinically. Hexaminolevulinate is the more potent analog, with greater local bioavailability and superior fluorescence intensity, and is approved for single clinical use in Europe and the United States for patients with suspected or known bladder cancer. Owing to a false-positive fluorescence from inflammatory lesions, previous biopsy sites, or in patients previously treated with bacillus Calmette-Guérin,[7,19] hexaminolevulinate is not approved currently for patients who received intravesical immunotherapy or chemotherapy within 90 days.

Multi-institutional, randomized, clinical studies have demonstrated that PDD improves the detection of papillary bladder tumors.[19,20] Although PDD does not distinguish high-grade from low-grade bladder cancer, several studies have shown that PDD has an increased rate of detection of flat-appearing CIS.[19,20] In a meta-analysis of 3 phase III studies, the detection of CIS was significantly higher by PDD plus WLC compared with WLC alone (87% vs 75% pooled sensitivity; $P = .006$).[21] Additionally, several meta-analyses have found significantly reduced residual tumor rates in patients treated with PDD, with relative risk of residual tumor 2.77-fold higher for WLC compared with PDD.[22,23]

The recurrence rate of PDD-guided TUR of bladder tumor remains to be determined. In a meta-analysis that reviewed raw data from prospective studies on 1345 patients with known or suspected non–muscle-invasive bladder cancer, overall recurrence rates up to 12 months were significantly lower with PDD compared with WLC (34.5% vs 45.4% pooled sensitivity; $P = .006$) and independent of the level of risk.[24] However, a prospective randomized multi-institutional trial found no difference in tumor recurrence and progression between PDD and WLC in patients with non–muscle-invasive bladder cancer.[25] Additional studies with longer follow-up time periods are needed to better define the optimal indications for PDD use and evaluate the long-term efficacy of PDD with regard to recurrence-free and progression-free survival.

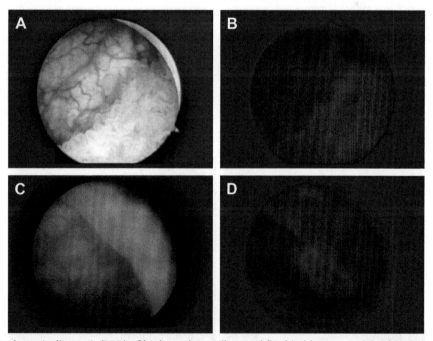

Fig. 1. Photodynamic diagnosis (PDD) of high-grade papillary and flat bladder cancer. (*A*) White light cystoscopy (WLC) showed a large broad-based papillary tumor. (*B*) PDD showed diffuse pink fluorescence over the tumor. Subsequent pathology for the lesion imaged in (*A*) and (*B*) confirmed noninvasive high-grade urothelial carcinoma. In a different patient, (*C*) WLC showed minimal erythema on the bladder mucosa along the left lateral wall; however, (*D*) PDD showed a pink fluorescence over the region that was confirmed to be noninvasive high-grade urothelial carcinoma and carcinoma in situ on histopathology.

NARROW BAND IMAGING

NBI is a high-resolution wide-field endoscopic technique that improves detection of bladder neoplasia through enhanced visualization of mucosal and submucosal vasculature without the use of exogenous dye. NBI devices (Olympus Corp, Tokyo, Japan) filter out the red spectrum from white light, with the resultant blue (415 nm) and green (540 nm) spectra absorbed by hemoglobin, thus highlighting the contrast between capillaries and mucosa. Under NBI, the more vascularized CIS or tumor areas are accentuated in appearance as green or brown (**Fig. 2**). NBI is approved for clinical use in the United States and is available either in an integrated videocystoscope or through a camera head that can be attached to standard cystoscopes. These devices include a toggling functionality between WLC and NBI, thereby facilitating rapid and real-time evaluation of suspected lesions. Although NBI provides a subjective impression of abnormal areas of bladder mucosa, there does not seem to be a significant difference in detection rate of bladder tumor between new and experienced users.[26,27]

In a recent meta-analysis of 8 studies including 1022 patients, the detection of bladder cancer was higher by NBI compared with WLC on a per-person basis (94% vs 85% pooled sensitivity) and a per-lesion basis (95% vs 75% pooled sensitivity); however, the pooled specificity on a per-lesion basis was lower by NBI compared with WLC (55% vs 72%).[28]

Similar to PDD, NBI does not distinguish bladder cancer grade, but does improve CIS detection. In a study of 427 patients that compared NBI plus WLC with WLC alone for recurrent bladder cancer, the detection of CIS was significantly improved by NBI over WLC (100% vs 83% sensitivity).[29] A single-center, prospective, randomized, controlled trial involving 220 patients with bulky non–muscle-invasive bladder tumor demonstrated an improved detection rate of CIS for NBI compared with WLC (95% vs 68%).[30] A multicenter, prospective study reported a significantly increased sensitivity for the detection of CIS from 50% for WLC to 90% for NBI in 104 patients.[31]

In a recent, single-center, randomized, controlled trial to assess whether NBI improved TUR of bladder tumors in 254 patients with 2-year follow-up, a reduced recurrence rate (22% vs 33%; $P = .05$) and improved recurrence-free survival (22 vs 19 months; $P = .02$) were reported by NBI compared with WLC.[32] A multicenter, randomized, controlled trial to compare the recurrence rate at 1 year between NBI- and WLC-assisted TUR of bladder tumor in patients with non–muscle-invasive bladder cancer is ongoing.[33]

CONFOCAL LASER ENDOMICROSCOPY

CLE is an optical biopsy technology that provides dynamic, high-resolution microscopy of mucosal lesions.[34] Recently approved for clinical use in the urinary tract, image acquisition is performed through fiber optic probes ranging from 0.85 to 2.6 mm in diameter, compatible with working channels of standard cystoscopes.[35] Fluorescein, a US Food and Drug Administration–approved drug, is used as the contrast agent and can be administered intravesically or intravenously with minimal toxicity.[36] In the current CLE clinical system (Mauna Kea Technologies, Paris, France), illuminating light from a 488-nm laser fiber source is focused by an objective lens, with scattered light from the in-focus tissue plane converged back

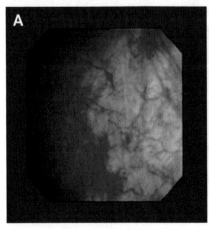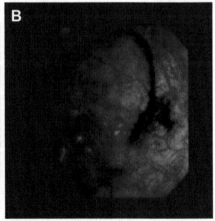

Fig. 2. Narrow band imaging (NBI) of the bladder. (*A*) White light cystoscopy of the left lateral wall regions showed only mild erythema. (*B*) Under NBI, brown fluorescence delineated the extent of more vascularized neoplastic areas, subsequently confirmed on pathology to be high-grade noninvasive urothelial carcinoma.

into the fiber and subsequent signal processing into an image. CLE provides the highest spatial resolution (1–5 μm) of clinically available technologies, with images comparable with conventional histopathology. Video sequences are acquiring at 12 frames per second, allowing for real-time dynamic imaging of physiologic processes such as vascular flow.

Given spatial resolution sufficient to resolve microarchitectural and cellular features, CLE is capable of differentiating high-grade and low-grade bladder cancer. After the initial pilot study that demonstrated the feasibility of using CLE in ex vivo bladders after cystectomy,[37] CLE was conducted in 27 patients undergoing cystoscopy and TUR and differences between normal urothelium, low-grade tumors and high-grade tumors were visualized.[34] In normal urothelium, larger umbrella cells were seen most superficially followed by organized smaller intermediate cells with distinct cell borders. Low-grade papillary tumors demonstrated densely arranged but normal-shaped small cells extending outward from fibrovascular cores, whereas high-grade tumors and CIS showed markedly irregular architecture and cellular pleomorphism (**Fig. 3**).

An imaging atlas based on 66 patients has been created to establish criteria for CLE diagnosis and grading of bladder cancer.[38] A recent study that analyzed 31 bladder regions with CLE and WLC demonstrated moderate interobserver agreement in image interpretation between novice and experienced CLE urologists with respect to cancer diagnosis; interestingly, experienced CLE urologists were found to have higher agreement for image interpretation with CLE compared with WLC alone (90% vs 74%).[39] Multicenter studies examining the diagnostic accuracy of CLE for real-time cancer diagnosis and grading remain to be completed.

OPTICAL COHERENCE TOMOGRAPHY

OCT is another optical biopsy technology that provides high-resolution, real-time, subsurface imaging of tissues. Analogous to B-mode ultrasonography, OCT relies on information gathered by reflected energy. Unlike ultrasonography, however, OCT utilizes near-infrared light (890–1300 nm) and measures the backscatter properties of different tissue layers to provide a cross-sectional image with 2 mm depth of penetration and 10 to 20 μm spatial resolution.[40] Under OCT, normal urothelium is seen as a weakly scattering darker layer, the lamina propria is a bright layer with the highest scattering intensity, and the muscularis propria is a less scattering layer beneath the lamina propria. In cancerous tissue, anatomic layers of the

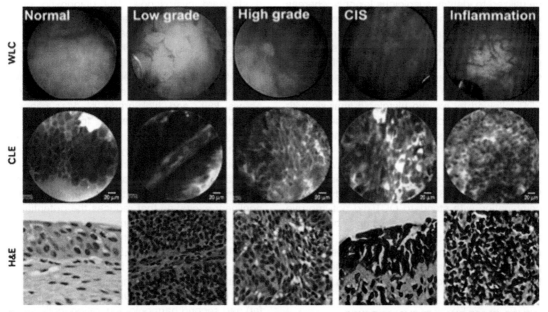

Fig. 3. Optical biopsy of the bladder using confocal laser endomicroscopy (CLE). Normal, low-grade, high-grade papillary bladder cancer, carcinoma in situ (CIS), and inflammation CLE images are shown with corresponding WLC images and hematoxylin and eosin (H&E) staining from subsequent biopsy. Low-grade cancer shows characteristically organized papillary structures, in contrast with high-grade cancer and CIS that display pleomorphic cells and distorted microarchitecture. (*From* Hsu M, Gupta M, Su LM, et al. Intraoperative optical imaging and tissue interrogation during urologic surgery. Curr Opin Urol 2014;24:66; with permission.)

urothelium are lost.[41,42] Limitations of OCT include false-positive results, possibly owing to disruptions of the bladder wall from erosion, scarring, or granuloma formation.[40,43]

Multiple studies have evaluated the real-time classification by OCT-assisted cystoscopy of bladder lesions as benign or malignant, with overall sensitivity 84% to 100% and overall specificity 65% to 89%.[40,43–47] Although OCT does not distinguish neoplastic bladder lesions by tumor grade, it is the only optical imaging technology with sufficient subsurface tissue penetration for real-time assessment of invasiveness of bladder lesions (ie, staging).[43–45] In a single-center study involving 24 patients at high risk for bladder cancer, the positive predictive value for tumor invasion into the lamina propria diagnosed by OCT was 90%.[40] Other recent studies have reported an automated image-processing algorithm to detect bladder cancer from OCT images[48] and application in the upper tract.[49] Larger multicenter studies are needed to evaluate the diagnostic value of tumor invasion by OCT as an adjunct to cytology, WLC, and histopathology.

MULTIMODAL IMAGING

The combination of imaging modalities harbors the potential to increase diagnostic accuracy. For example, macroscopic imaging (PDD, NBI) could be utilized to identify suspicious lesions, whereas microscopic imaging (CLE, OCT) could provide grading or staging information via high-resolution tissue characterization.[7,50] A recent study reported the feasibility of simultaneous PDD and CLE; however, intraoperative tumor grading was not done because TUR was performed using PDD followed by ex vivo histologic analysis with CLE.[51] Another study evaluated 232 lesions from 66 patients with suspected bladder cancer using WLC, PDD alone, and PDD plus OCT.[52] The combination of PDD and OCT compared with PDD alone significantly increased per-patient specificity from 62% to 87%. In another study, PDD in combination with standard OCT did not improve diagnostic accuracy in detecting noninvasive bladder cancer, but the combined use of cross-polarization OCT and PDD improved the positive predictive and negative predictive values in detecting bladder cancer in flat suspicious areas.[53]

OTHER EMERGING TECHNOLOGIES

In addition to these modalities, a number of emerging technologies are at advanced prototype phase or early clinical feasibility stage. Raman spectroscopy is based on the principle of scattering of photons following interaction with molecular bonds. As near infrared light (785–845 nm) illuminates the tissue, the donation of energy to molecular bonds results in a different wavelength of the photons exiting the sample (Raman shift).[54] Detection of these scattered photons is then plotted to create a spectrum of peaks, producing a molecular "fingerprint" of the examined sample without the requirement of an exogenous contrast agent.[55] In the ex vivo setting, Raman spectroscopy has been shown to differentiate the normal bladder wall layers, assess invasiveness, and identify low- and high-grade bladder cancers.[56,57] The first in vivo study utilized a Raman probe compatible with endoscopic working channels and reported sensitivity of 85% and specificity of 79% for the detection of bladder cancer in 62 suspected lesions.[55] Surface-enhanced Raman scattering nanoparticles have been shown to augment weak signals and allow for conjugation to cancer-specific antibodies to enable Raman-based molecular imaging.[58]

Ultraviolet (UV) autofluorescence is based on the UV laser excitation of the fluorescence of molecules naturally present in tissue. A recent pilot in vivo study compared spectroscopic results with histologic findings in 14 patients who underwent cystoscopy.[59] Normal urothelium, papillary tumors, and suspicious flat lesions were interrogated with a UV probe via the working channel of a standard cystoscope. The diagnostic signal was then converted into an intensity ratio of the emitted light at approximately 360 and 450 nm and color coded to facilitate real-time interpretation.[59] Differentiation of bladder cancer from normal urothelium was demonstrated. Additional studies are required to investigate signal intensity across low- and high-grade bladder cancers, reproducibility, and potential for UV-induced toxicity.

Multiphoton microscopy (MPM) is a laser-scanning microscopy technique based on the simultaneous absorption of 2 (or 3) near-infrared photons (700–800 nm) to cause a localized nonlinear excitation that reduces the potential for cellular damage. MPM enables imaging of unstained tissue at submicron resolution in 3 dimensions to a depth of up to 0.5 mm by using intrinsic tissue emissions signals from autofluorescence (nicotinamide adenine dinucleotide hydrogen in cells, elastin in connective tissue, lipofuscin in fat) and second harmonic generation (collagen).[60] The interpretation of acquired images is simplified by color coding the detected signals. A recent in vitro study reported MPM imaging on 77 fresh bladder biopsies, with 88% accuracy in differentiation between benign and neoplastic lesions and

68% accuracy in the assignment of cytologic grading.[61] Similar to CLE, limitations of MPM include limited depth of penetration that is not sufficient for cancer staging and a lack of nuclear detail. Current research is focused on the minituarization of the MPM system for in vivo application.[62,63]

Scanning fiber endoscopy (SFE) is an ultrathin flexible endoscope containing an optical fiber to provide wide-angle, full-color, high-resolution images.[64,65] The 1.2-mm diameter of the probe decreases invasiveness and allows versatility of use as either a standalone miniaturized endoscope or as a probe in conjunction with other imaging modalities.[66] SFE has been demonstrated in ex vivo bladder models.[67] Additional studies are required to investigate the feasibility of in vivo SFE. A potential application of SFE involves automated integration with an "image stitching" algorithm to generate a panoramic view of the urothelium that could be used for tumor mapping and surveying the bladder longitudinally.[67]

MOLECULAR IMAGING

Molecular imaging is the visualization and characterization of biologic processes at the molecular and cellular levels.[68] Molecular specificity may be conferred through coupling of optical imaging technologies with fluorescently labeled binding

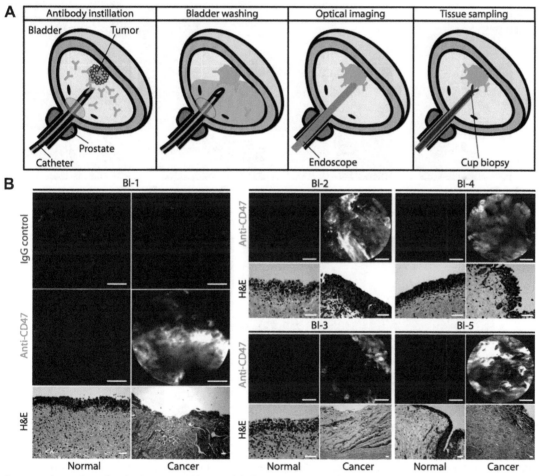

Fig. 4. Endoscopic molecular imaging of human bladder cancer using fluorescein labeled anti-CD47 as the imaging agent and confocal laser endomicroscopy (CLE) as the imaging modality. (*A*) Immediately after radical cystectomy, the ex vivo intact bladder was instilled with the molecular imaging agent via a urinary catheter and incubated for 30 minutes to allow antibody binding. After irrigation with saline, bound anti-CD47 was detected by endoscopic imaging of the bladder mucosa and normal and suspicious regions were biopsied for histopathologic analysis. (*B*) Representative frames of CLE videos acquired from normal and cancer lesions in 5 bladders (BI) with corresponding hematoxylin and eosin (H&E)–stained images. Scale bars, 50 mm. IgG, immunoglobulin G. (*From* Pan Y, Volkmer JP, Mach KE, et al. Endoscopic molecular imaging of human bladder cancer using a CD47 antibody. Sci Transl Med 2014;6:260ra148; with permission.)

agents such as antibodies, peptides, or small molecules. Bladder, given the ease of access and an established track record of intravesical therapy, is a promising target organ for endoscopic molecular imaging. Fluorescently labeled, cancer-specific molecular imaging agents may provide enhanced differentiation between tumor and adjacent normal or benign tissues. Thus, the combination of optical imaging technologies with cancer-specific molecular imaging agents holds the potential for real-time endoscopic cancer detection.[69,70]

A recent study used fluorescently labeled CD47 antibody (anti-CD47) to successfully demonstrate ex vivo endoscopic molecular imaging of bladder cancer using CLE and PDD in 25 intact bladders derived from radical cystectomy.[71] All of the bladders were derived from patients with invasive high-grade bladder cancer. CD47 is a surface marker of human solid tumors and is expressed on more than 80% of bladder cancer cells.[72,73] A monoclonal CD47 antibody under development as a targeted therapy agent was labeled with a

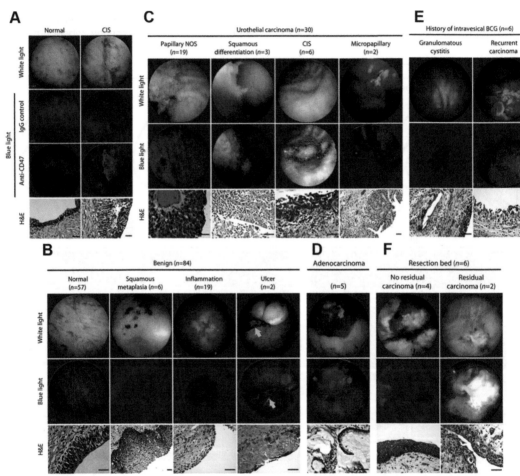

Fig. 5. Endoscopic molecular imaging of human bladder cancer using anti–CD47-labeled with a quantum dot nanocrystal (Qdot$_{625}$) and imaged with blue light cystoscope from a clinical photodynamic diagnosis (PDD) system. Representative white light cystoscopy (WLC) and PDD images with corresponding hematoxylin and eosin (H&E) staining for colocalization of anti–CD47-Qdot$_{625}$ binding and histopathology. (A) Cancer-specific binding of anti-CD47-Qdot$_{625}$ in a bladder with normal mucosa and a carcinoma in situ (CIS) lesion. (B) Benign regions of normal urothelium, squamous metaplasia, inflammation, and ulcer (arrows) with no detectable anti–CD47-Qdot$_{625}$ binding. (C) Anti–CD47-Qdot$_{625}$ binding detected under PDD on urothelial carcinomas. (D) Anti–CD47-Qdot$_{625}$ bound to adenocarcinoma of the bladder. (E) In a bladder with a history of bacillus Calmette-Guérin (BCG) treatment, anti–CD47-Qdot$_{625}$ bound to a region with recurrent carcinoma but did not bind to a region of cystitis. (F) Anti–CD47-Qdot$_{625}$ bound to residual tumor in a prior resection bed but not to benign scar tissue. Scale bars, 50 mm. IgG, immunoglobulin G; NOS, not otherwise specified. (Adapted from Pan Y, Volkmer JP, Mach KE, et al. Endoscopic molecular imaging of human bladder cancer using a CD47 antibody. Sci Transl Med 2014;6:260ra148; with permission.)

fluorescent tag, either fluorescein isothiocyanate (FITC) or quantum dot, a semiconductor nanocrystal, was instilled intravesically as a topical molecular imaging agent (**Fig. 4**A). After allowing sufficient time for antibody binding, excess antibody was removed by bladder irrigation. Bladders incubated with anti-CD47–FITC were imaged with CLE (see **Fig. 4**B) and those incubated with anti–CD47-$Qdot_{625}$ were imaged by PDD (**Fig. 5**). In all bladders imaged with CLE, anti-CD47–FITC binding to cancer lesions was between 95- and 1100-fold greater than binding to normal urothelium in the same bladder. In the bladders imaged with PDD, the sensitivity and specificity for CD47-targeted imaging were 82.9% and 90.5%, respectively, indicating the potential of CD47 to serve as a bladder cancer imaging agent with improved disease specificity. Further studies to assess the in vivo binding and toxicity of labeled anti-CD47 will be required before clinical translation. The study offers the promising possibility that targeted therapy may be combined with targeted imaging.

SUMMARY

New optical imaging technologies have emerged and hold the potential to revolutionize the detection and management of bladder cancer beyond WLC. Macroscopic technologies such as PDD and NBI improve the detection of bladder cancer and are already implemented in the clinical setting. Microscopic technologies such as OCT and CLE provide optical biopsy techniques that enable subsurface imaging comparable with standard histopathology. CLE is the only clinically available imaging technique capable of differentiating between low-grade and high-grade bladder cancers. Molecular imaging represents an exciting innovation that combines optical imaging technologies with cancer-specific molecular agents to improve the specificity of disease detection and potentially grading differentiation. Additional studies are needed to further define the role of imaging technologies in the evaluation and management of high-grade bladder cancer.

REFERENCES

1. Siegel R, Ma J, Zou Z, et al. Cancer statistics, 2014. CA Cancer J Clin 2014;64:9.
2. Kirkali Z, Chan T, Manoharan M, et al. Bladder cancer: epidemiology, staging and grading, and diagnosis. Urology 2005;66:4.
3. Morgan TM, Keegan KA, Clark PE. Bladder cancer. Curr Opin Oncol 2011;23:275.
4. Sylvester RJ, van der Meijden AP, Oosterlinck W, et al. Predicting recurrence and progression in individual patients with stage Ta T1 bladder cancer using EORTC risk tables: a combined analysis of 2596 patients from seven EORTC trials. Eur Urol 2006;49:466.
5. Avritscher EB, Cooksley CD, Grossman HB, et al. Clinical model of lifetime cost of treating bladder cancer and associated complications. Urology 2006;68:549.
6. Lee CS, Yoon CY, Witjes JA. The past, present and future of cystoscopy: the fusion of cystoscopy and novel imaging technology. BJU Int 2008;102:1228.
7. Liu JJ, Droller MJ, Liao JC. New optical imaging technologies for bladder cancer: considerations and perspectives. J Urol 2012;188:361.
8. Cina SJ, Epstein JI, Endrizzi JM, et al. Correlation of cystoscopic impression with histologic diagnosis of biopsy specimens of the bladder. Hum Pathol 2001;32:630.
9. Fradet Y, Grossman HB, Gomella L, et al. A comparison of hexaminolevulinate fluorescence cystoscopy and white light cystoscopy for the detection of carcinoma in situ in patients with bladder cancer: a phase III, multicenter study. J Urol 2007;178:68.
10. Jocham D, Witjes F, Wagner S, et al. Improved detection and treatment of bladder cancer using hexaminolevulinate imaging: a prospective, phase III multicenter study. J Urol 2005;174:862.
11. Schmidbauer J, Witjes F, Schmeller N, et al. Improved detection of urothelial carcinoma in situ with hexaminolevulinate fluorescence cystoscopy. J Urol 2004;171:135.
12. Babjuk M, Soukup V, Petrik R, et al. 5-aminolaevulinic acid-induced fluorescence cystoscopy during transurethral resection reduces the risk of recurrence in stage Ta/T1 bladder cancer. BJU Int 2005; 96:798.
13. Daniltchenko DI, Riedl CR, Sachs MD, et al. Long-term benefit of 5-aminolevulinic acid fluorescence assisted transurethral resection of superficial bladder cancer: 5-year results of a prospective randomized study. J Urol 2005;174:2129.
14. Kolozsy Z. Histopathological "self control" in transurethral resection of bladder tumours. Br J Urol 1991;67:162.
15. Cheng L, Neumann RM, Weaver AL, et al. Grading and staging of bladder carcinoma in transurethral resection specimens. Correlation with 105 matched cystectomy specimens. Am J Clin Pathol 2000;113: 275.
16. Brausi M, Collette L, Kurth K, et al. Variability in the recurrence rate at first follow-up cystoscopy after TUR in stage Ta T1 transitional cell carcinoma of the bladder: a combined analysis of seven EORTC studies. Eur Urol 2002;41:523.
17. Klan R, Loy V, Huland H. Residual tumor discovered in routine second transurethral resection in patients

with stage T1 transitional cell carcinoma of the bladder. J Urol 1991;146:316.

18. Mark JR, Gelpi-Hammerschmidt F, Trabulsi EJ, et al. Blue light cystoscopy for detection and treatment of non-muscle invasive bladder cancer. Can J Urol 2012;19:6227.

19. Lapini A, Minervini A, Masala A, et al. A comparison of hexaminolevulinate (Hexvix((R))) fluorescence cystoscopy and white-light cystoscopy for detection of bladder cancer: results of the HeRo observational study. Surg Endosc 2012;26:3634.

20. Rink M, Babjuk M, Catto JW, et al. Hexyl aminolevulinate-guided fluorescence cystoscopy in the diagnosis and follow-up of patients with non-muscle-invasive bladder cancer: a critical review of the current literature. Eur Urol 2013;64:624.

21. Lerner SP, Liu H, Wu MF, et al. Fluorescence and white light cystoscopy for detection of carcinoma in situ of the urinary bladder. Urol Oncol 2012;30:285.

22. Shen P, Yang J, Wei W, et al. Effects of fluorescent light-guided transurethral resection on non-muscle-invasive bladder cancer: a systematic review and meta-analysis. BJU Int 2012;110:E209.

23. Kausch I, Sommerauer M, Montorsi F, et al. Photodynamic diagnosis in non-muscle-invasive bladder cancer: a systematic review and cumulative analysis of prospective studies. Eur Urol 2010;57:595.

24. Burger M, Grossman HB, Droller M, et al. Photodynamic diagnosis of non-muscle-invasive bladder cancer with hexaminolevulinate cystoscopy: a meta-analysis of detection and recurrence based on raw data. Eur Urol 2013;64:846.

25. Schumacher MC, Holmang S, Davidsson T, et al. Transurethral resection of non-muscle-invasive bladder transitional cell cancers with or without 5-aminolevulinic Acid under visible and fluorescent light: results of a prospective, randomised, multi-centre study. Eur Urol 2010;57:293.

26. Bryan RT, Shah ZH, Collins SI, et al. Narrow-band imaging flexible cystoscopy: a new user's experience. J Endourol 2010;24:1339.

27. Herr H, Donat M, Dalbagni G, et al. Narrow-band imaging cystoscopy to evaluate bladder tumours–individual surgeon variability. BJU Int 2010;106:53.

28. Zheng C, Lv Y, Zhong Q, et al. Narrow band imaging diagnosis of bladder cancer: systematic review and meta-analysis. BJU Int 2012;110:E680.

29. Herr HW, Donat SM. A comparison of white-light cystoscopy and narrow-band imaging cystoscopy to detect bladder tumour recurrences. BJU Int 2008;102:1111.

30. Geavlete B, Multescu R, Georgescu D, et al. Narrow band imaging cystoscopy and bipolar plasma vaporization for large nonmuscle-invasive bladder tumors–results of a prospective, randomized comparison to the standard approach. Urology 2012;79:846.

31. Tatsugami K, Kuroiwa K, Kamoto T, et al. Evaluation of narrow-band imaging as a complementary method for the detection of bladder cancer. J Endourol 1807;24:2010.

32. Herr HW. Randomized trial of narrow-band versus white-light cystoscopy for restaging (second-look) transurethral resection of bladder tumors. Eur Urol 2015;67:605–8.

33. Naito S, van Rees Vellinga S, de la Rosette J. Global randomized narrow band imaging versus white light study in nonmuscle invasive bladder cancer: accession to the first milestone-enrollment of 600 patients. J Endourol 2013;27:1.

34. Sonn GA, Jones SN, Tarin TV, et al. Optical biopsy of human bladder neoplasia with in vivo confocal laser endomicroscopy. J Urol 2009;182:1299.

35. Adams W, Wu K, Liu JJ, et al. Comparison of 2.6- and 1.4-mm imaging probes for confocal laser endomicroscopy of the urinary tract. J Endourol 2011;25:917.

36. Wallace MB, Meining A, Canto MI, et al. The safety of intravenous fluorescein for confocal laser endomicroscopy in the gastrointestinal tract. Aliment Pharmacol Ther 2010;31:548.

37. Sonn GA, Mach KE, Jensen K, et al. Fibered confocal microscopy of bladder tumors: an ex vivo study. J Endourol 2009;23:197.

38. Wu K, Liu JJ, Adams W, et al. Dynamic real-time microscopy of the urinary tract using confocal laser endomicroscopy. Urology 2011;78:225.

39. Chang TC, Liu JJ, Hsiao ST, et al. Interobserver agreement of confocal laser endomicroscopy for bladder cancer. J Endourol 2013;27:598.

40. Manyak MJ, Gladkova ND, Makari JH, et al. Evaluation of superficial bladder transitional-cell carcinoma by optical coherence tomography. J Endourol 2005;19:570.

41. Zagaynova EV, Streltsova OS, Gladkova ND, et al. In vivo optical coherence tomography feasibility for bladder disease. J Urol 2002;167:1492.

42. Sergeev A, Gelikonov V, Gelikonov G, et al. In vivo endoscopic OCT imaging of precancer and cancer states of human mucosa. Opt Express 1997;1:432.

43. Goh AC, Tresser NJ, Shen SS, et al. Optical coherence tomography as an adjunct to white light cystoscopy for intravesical real-time imaging and staging of bladder cancer. Urology 2008;72:133.

44. Hermes B, Spoler F, Naami A, et al. Visualization of the basement membrane zone of the bladder by optical coherence tomography: feasibility of noninvasive evaluation of tumor invasion. Urology 2008;72:677.

45. Karl A, Stepp H, Willmann E, et al. Optical coherence tomography for bladder cancer – ready as a surrogate for optical biopsy? Results of a prospective mono-centre study. Eur J Med Res 2010;15:131.

46. Ren H, Waltzer WC, Bhalla R, et al. Diagnosis of bladder cancer with microelectromechanical

systems-based cystoscopic optical coherence tomography. Urology 2009;74:1351.

47. Sengottayan VK, Vasudeva P, Dalela D. Intravesical real-time imaging and staging of bladder cancer: use of optical coherence tomography. Indian J Urol 2008;24:592.

48. Lingley-Papadopoulos CA, Loew MH, Manyak MJ, et al. Computer recognition of cancer in the urinary bladder using optical coherence tomography and texture analysis. J Biomed Opt 2008;13:024003.

49. Bus MT, Muller BG, de Bruin DM, et al. Volumetric in vivo visualization of upper urinary tract tumors using optical coherence tomography: a pilot study. J Urol 2013;190:2236.

50. Lopez A, Liao JC. Emerging endoscopic imaging technologies for bladder cancer detection. Curr Urol Rep 2014;15:406.

51. Bonnal JL, Rock A Jr, Gagnat A, et al. Confocal laser endomicroscopy of bladder tumors associated with photodynamic diagnosis: an ex vivo pilot study. Urology 2012;80:1162.e1.

52. Schmidbauer J, Remzi M, Klatte T, et al. Fluorescence cystoscopy with high-resolution optical coherence tomography imaging as an adjunct reduces false-positive findings in the diagnosis of urothelial carcinoma of the bladder. Eur Urol 2009;56:914.

53. Gladkova N, Kiseleva E, Streltsova O, et al. Combined use of fluorescence cystoscopy and cross-polarization OCT for diagnosis of bladder cancer and correlation with immunohistochemical markers. J Biophotonics 2013;6:687.

54. Rao AR, Hanchanale V, Javle P, et al. Spectroscopic view of life and work of the Nobel Laureate Sir C.V. Raman. J Endourol 2007;21:8.

55. Draga RO, Grimbergen MC, Vijverberg PL, et al. In vivo bladder cancer diagnosis by high-volume Raman spectroscopy. Anal Chem 2010;82:5993.

56. Crow P, Uff JS, Farmer JA, et al. The use of Raman spectroscopy to identify and characterize transitional cell carcinoma in vitro. BJU Int 2004;93:1232.

57. de Jong BW, Bakker Schut TC, Wolffenbuttel KP, et al. Identification of bladder wall layers by Raman spectroscopy. J Urol 2002;168:1771.

58. Vendrell M, Maiti KK, Dhaliwal K, et al. Surface-enhanced Raman scattering in cancer detection and imaging. Trends Biotechnol 2013;31:249.

59. Schafauer C, Ettori D, Roupret M, et al. Detection of bladder urothelial carcinoma using in vivo noncontact, ultraviolet excited autofluorescence measurements converted into simple color coded images: a feasibility study. J Urol 2013;190:271.

60. Zipfel WR, Williams RM, Webb WW. Nonlinear magic: multiphoton microscopy in the biosciences. Nat Biotechnol 2003;21:1369.

61. Jain M, Robinson BD, Scherr DS, et al. Multiphoton microscopy in the evaluation of human bladder biopsies. Arch Pathol Lab Med 2012;136:517.

62. Rivera DR, Brown CM, Ouzounov DG, et al. Compact and flexible raster scanning multiphoton endoscope capable of imaging unstained tissue. Proc Natl Acad Sci U S A 2011;108:17598.

63. Tewari AK, Shevchuk MM, Sterling J, et al. Multiphoton microscopy for structure identification in human prostate and periprostatic tissue: implications in prostate cancer surgery. BJU Int 2011;108:1421.

64. Seibel EJ, Brentnall TA, Dominitz JA. New endoscopic and cytologic tools for cancer surveillance in the digestive tract. Gastrointest Endosc Clin N Am 2009;19:299.

65. Seibel EJ, Brown CM, Dominitz JA, et al. Scanning single fiber endoscopy: a new platform technology for integrated laser imaging, diagnosis, and future therapies. Gastrointest Endosc Clin N Am 2008;18:467.

66. Yoon WJ, Park S, Reinhall PG, et al. Development of an Automated Steering Mechanism for Bladder Urothelium Surveillance. J Med Device 2009;3:11004.

67. Soper TD, Porter MP, Seibel EJ. Surface mosaics of the bladder reconstructed from endoscopic video for automated surveillance. IEEE Trans Biomed Eng 2012;59:1670.

68. Greco F, Cadeddu JA, Gill IS, et al. Current perspectives in the use of molecular imaging to target surgical treatments for genitourinary cancers. Eur Urol 2014;65:947.

69. van Dam GM, Themelis G, Crane LM, et al. Intraoperative tumor-specific fluorescence imaging in ovarian cancer by folate receptor-alpha targeting: first in-human results. Nat Med 2011;17:1315.

70. Nguyen QT, Tsien RY. Fluorescence-guided surgery with live molecular navigation–a new cutting edge. Nat Rev Cancer 2013;13:653.

71. Pan Y, Volkmer JP, Mach KE, et al. Endoscopic molecular imaging of human bladder cancer using a CD47 antibody. Sci Transl Med 2014;6:260ra148.

72. Chan KS, Espinosa I, Chao M, et al. Identification, molecular characterization, clinical prognosis, and therapeutic targeting of human bladder tumor-initiating cells. Proc Natl Acad Sci U S A 2009;106:14016.

73. Willingham SB, Volkmer JP, Gentles AJ, et al. The CD47-signal regulatory protein alpha (SIRPa) interaction is a therapeutic target for human solid tumors. Proc Natl Acad Sci U S A 2012;109:6662.

Novel Therapeutic Approaches for Recurrent Nonmuscle Invasive Bladder Cancer

Brock E. Boehm, DO, Robert S. Svatek, MD, MSCI*

KEYWORDS

- Bladder • Cancer • Novel • Therapeutics

KEY POINTS

- Pharmacokinetics of intravesical chemotherapy delivery demonstrates that treatment of bladder cancer cells located deep to the superficial cell layer is inadequate.
- BCG vaccine's clinical activity is thought to depend in part on eliciting a Th1 immune responses characterized by increases in pro-inflammatory cytokines such as interleukin (IL)-2 and interferon (INF-γ).
- Checkpoint inhibitors, including programmed death-1 (PD-1) and programmed death ligand 1 inhibitors, have demonstrated impressive and durable antitumor response in advanced, metastatic bladder cancer, and this has prompted considerations for testing in nonmuscle invasive bladder cancer.

INTRODUCTION

Urothelial cell carcinoma of the bladder is the fourth most common malignancy in men, and most present with nonmuscle invasive bladder cancer (NMIBC). It is currently estimated there will be 74,690 new cases of bladder cancer in the United States, with 15,580 estimated deaths in 2014.[1] Standard therapy for NMIBC is complete transurethral resection of the bladder tumor (TURBT). In some cases, perioperative or adjuvant intravesical therapy is indicated. Bacillus Calmette-Guérin (BCG) immunotherapy is indicated for high-grade disease, and this has been the stable of standard care since it received US Food and Drug Administration (FDA) approval for the treatment and prophylaxis of NMIBC. Despite the success of BCG therapy, however, recurrence rates remain high, and progression is still possible.[2] Patients who fail BCG therapy have limited options, and most will succumb to bladder removal. Thus, there is strong impetus to find alternative treatment options in NMIBC.

This article aims to provide a summary of novel strategies currently being investigated in patients with NMIBC. It focuses on approaches that have initiated studies in patients, including phase 1 through 3 trials and pilot studies. Considerable progress has been made toward improving the delivery method of the available intravesical agents. Presently, intravesical therapy is limited by the finite amount of time that the agent remains in contact with the bladder. Bladder cancer is widely considered to be responsive to immune therapy, as BCG immunotherapy has been the mainstay of treatment for decades. Thus, many novel approaches are immune-based therapies and include cancer vaccines, use of BCG subcomponents, and checkpoint inhibitors. Finally, access to bladder mucosa via direct catheterization into

Disclosures: There are no financial disclosures.
Adult Cancer Program, Department of Urology, Cancer Therapy and Research Center, The University of Texas Health Science Center San Antonio, 7703 Floyd Curl Drive, San Antonio, TX 78023, USA
* Corresponding author.
E-mail address: svatek@uthscsa.edu

Urol Clin N Am 42 (2015) 159–168
http://dx.doi.org/10.1016/j.ucl.2015.02.001

the bladder via the urethra has enabled unique strategies for delivery of cancer therapy including viral- or plasmid-based gene therapy. These and other miscellaneous approaches currently being developed for testing in patients with NMIBC will be reviewed. Current therapeutic trials in nonmuscle invasive bladder cancer accessed in clinicaltrials.gov are represented in (**Table 1**).

Delivery Methods

The structure of the urothelium and function of the bladder serve as a restrictive barrier that creates unique challenges when considering delivery of intravesical therapy. The bladder is constantly receiving urine, and as such, will begin to dilute the agent in question as urine is drained from the kidneys. It will also rapidly wash out the agent during the bladder's voiding stage.

The urothelium itself is composed of 3 distinct cell layers: superficial umbrella cells that measure 100 to 200 μm; intermediate cells (20 μm), and a basal cell layer (5–10 μm), which makes up a layer that functions as precursor stem cells and lies immediately superficial to the basement membrane.[3] On the apical surface of the umbrella cells lie several different glycosaminoglycans that act as a barrier to potential toxic substances that may be in the urine.[3] These hydrophilic molecules extend far above the cell surface and function to create an aqueous layer that serves as a barrier between the bladder lumen and urothelium.

Electromotive drug administration

Studies analyzing the pharmacokinetics of intravesical chemotherapy delivery noted that treatment of bladder cancer cells located deep to the superficial cell layer was inadequate.[4] This was thought to be secondary to decreased drug concentrations beyond the urothelium, and electromotive therapy was proposed as a means to improve drug penetration. When exposed to a conductive current such as NaCl and an electrical field, mitomycin (MMC) delivery across the urothelium increases as a result of current-induced convective flow of water. Thus, water will bring the nonionized MMC particle with it across the urothelium as it travels down its electrical gradient. Results indicated that mean concentration of MMC in the bladder wall delivered by electromotive drug administration vastly exceeded MMC concentration achieved through passive delivery by a factor of almost 7.[5]

In a randomized controlled trial of adjuvant treatment following complete transurethral resection, patients with T1 bladder cancer assigned sequential BCG and electromotive MMC had a longer disease-free interval than did those assigned BCG

alone.[6] However, because patients in the control group did not receive standard maintenance BCG therapy, the benefit of this therapy over standard BCG remains to be tested. More recently, benefit of electromotive therapy was also observed in the perioperative setting. In a phase 3 study enrolling patients with NMIBC, the efficacy of TURBT alone was compared with that of immediate post-TURBT passive diffusion MMC or immediate pre-TURBT electromotive MMC. With a median follow-up of over 7 years, disease-free rates were: 36%, 41%, and 62% of patients treated with TURBT alone, post-TURBT passive diffusion of MMC, and pre-TURBT electromotive administration of MMC, respectively. This represents a 21% absolute improvement in disease-free rate over passive diffusion.[7] Electromotive MMC is not currently approved by the FDA.

Nanoparticle-based therapy

Small molecule platform nanoparticles can be engineered to increase the drug contact time with the urothelium by functioning as controlled drug release systems. They are specifically created to have multiple functional groups (eg, albumin, amine, carboxyl, or sulfhydryl) that can interact with the urothelium in order to increase adhesion rates. Nanoparticle albumin-bound (NAB) agents are currently under clinical investigation. The addition of albumin is proposed to increase solubility and facilitate drug delivery to tumor cells through biological interactions with albumin receptors that facilitate drug transport across epithelial cells.[8] Intravesical administration of NAB linked with paclitaxel demonstrated safety and tolerability in a phase 1 trial including 18 patients with BCG-refractory high-grade Ta, T1, or carcinoma-in-situ (CIS).[9] Results of the phase 2 data were recently reported.[10] A complete response was observed in 10 (35.7%) of 28 patients treated with NAB-paclitaxel with recurrent NMIBC who had failed at least 1 prior BCG regimen.[10]

In murine models, the mTOR inhibitor rapamycin was found to potentiate the induction of BCG-mediated immune responses in mice.[11] In addition, rapamycin demonstrated antitumor activity in preclinical models of bladder cancer.[12] Albumin-bound rapamycin (ABI-009) could facilitate uptake of rapamycin, which is normally water-insoluble. This novel agent is currently being tested in early clinical trials for patients with BCG-refractory or recurrent NMIBC (NCT02009332).

Hydrogel formulations

One potential means to improve contact duration of intravesical therapy, including BCG, is through the use of a hydrogel delivery system. Thermosensitive hydrogels are able to exist as a free-flowing solution at room temperature, while becoming a viscous hydrogel at body temperature.[13] BCG introduced with this gel system could prove to be a valuable intravesical immunotherapeutic agent because of its ability to lead to sustained release of BCG as compared to the typical 2 hour duration witnessed in current BCG intravesical therapy delivery.[14] TC-3 is a hydrogel application currently under clinical investigation that uses a biodegradable gel, which remains in gel form to function as a drug reservoir inside the bladder, and dissolves when it comes in contact with the urine. A randomized trial of pre-TURBT administration is proposed to evaluate effects of MMC mixed with TC-3 gel on patients with papillary low risk recurrent NMIBC (NCT01803295).

Hyperthermia

Hyperthermia has been shown to increase urothelium penetration rate of immuno- and chemotherapeutic agents and has the potential to be an effective delivery method. Prospective cohort data from patients with NMIBC who had received prior intravesical therapy chemohyperthermia given by means of Synergo suggested that chemohyperthermia had potential to provide effective approach.[15] Patients underwent local microwave induced hyperthermia with a 915 MHz intravesical microwave applicator in addition to either MMC or epirubicin. While lacking a control group, an impressive 2-year disease-free interval of 47% and limited progression to muscle invasive disease (only 4%) among patients who had failed prior therapy was observed. Subsequently, intravesical thermochemotherapy by means of Synergo versus chemotherapy alone with MMC was tested in a randomized trial of 83 patients. Results demonstrated a 10-year disease free survival rate in the thermochemotherapy arm.[16] Further comparative trials are warranted, however, as less favorable results with significant adverse events have been described. In a report[17] of 21 patients treated with thermochemotherapy using Synergo, therapy was abandoned because of adverse effects in 38% of patients and there was limited tumor response.

Another heating device, the BSD-2000, was tested in a pilot study of patients with BCG refractory NMIBC. Fifteen patients were treated with external deep pelvic hyperthermia combined with MMC.[18] The bladders were heated to 42°C for 1 hour during intravesical MMC treatment. Full treatment course was attained in 73% of subjects and the device was deemed safe. Of note, heat-induced swelling of the abdominal skin was reported in 27% of patients.[18]

Hyaluronidase

Increased extracellular matrix deposition is a finding observed in various solid tumors. Increased levels of hyaluronan lead to decreased elasticity of tumor tissue. By hydrolyzing hyaluronan, hyaluronidase can increase permeability of chemotherapy into solid tumors. A phase I safety and tolerability study of immediate post-operative intravesical instillation of Chemophase is described for patients with any stage NMIBC (NCT00782587).[19] In this study, patients will be administered a single immediate post-operative intravesical instillation of recombinant human hyaluronidase in combination with mitomycin.

Gene Therapy

The bladder's anatomy and physiology give rise to a unique setting, one where immunotherapeutics and cytotoxics may be employed with minimal risk for systemic toxicity. In addition, the fact that the urethra also allows for ease of access to the urothelium for direct vector delivery, viral or plasma delivery systems for antineoplastics are currently being explored in several different studies.

Adenovirus CD40L

Adenovirus CD40L (AdCD40L) immunogene therapy for bladder cancer has undergone clinical testing. CD40 is a costimulatory protein found on antigen presenting cells such as dendritic cells. Binding of CD40 to CD40L, expressed on Th cells, activates the antigen-presenting cell. The proposed mechanism of action for this therapy is that increased expression of CD40L following adenoviral-mediated delivery disrupts tumor escape mechanisms, thereby allowing for improved tumor eradication in preclinical models.[20] In a clinical trial, 8 patients with Ta bladder cancer were treated with 3 cycles of weekly adCD40L therapy. The therapy was well tolerated, and gene transfer was detected through biopsied tissue.[21]

Recombinant adenovirus

The retinoblastoma tumor suppressor protein (RB) pathway is often deregulated in bladder cancer.[22] Recombinant adenovirus (CG0070) was developed to specifically target this pathway and facilitate precise antitumor activity. CG0070 is a replication selective serotype-5 oncolytic adenovirus that is able to lead to cancer-targeted replication and granulocyte macrophage-colony stimulating factor (GM-CSF) transgene expression.[23] This is accomplished through the E2F-1 promoter element, which in turn is regulated by RB, which aids in controlling viral replication rate as well as the expression of GM-CSF. GM-CSF is directly responsible for stimulating maturation

Table 1
Therapeutic trials in nonmuscle invasive bladder cancer accessed in Clinicaltrials.gov

Agent (ClinicalTrials.gov Identifier)	Setting	Population Studied	Method of Delivery
Delivery Methods			
EMDA-MMC (NCT01920269)	Adjuvant	Primary Ta-T1 and G1-2	Intravesical
EMDA-MMC (NCT02202044)	Adjuvant	Primary high-risk (Tis, G3 and/or T1 +/− concomitant Tis)	Intravesical
Albumin-bound rapamycin nanoparticles (NCT02009332)	Not specified	BCG refractory or recurrent Ta, T1, Tis	Intravesical
TC-3 Gel (NCT01803295)	Pre-TURBT	Low-risk recurrent (no high-grade, T1, Tis)	Intravesical
Hyperthermia-MMC (NCT01094964)	Adjuvant	BCG recurrent: Ta-1G2-3, concomitant Tis, or Tis alone	Intravesical
Chemophase (NCT00782587)	Within 6 h after TURBT	Ta, T1, or Tis of any grade	Intravesical
Gene Therapy			
CG0070 (NCT01438112)	Adjuvant	BCG refractory, high-grade (Ta-1 with concomitant Tis or Tis alone)	Intravesical
CG0070 (NCT02143804)	Adjuvant	BCG and NCT01438112 refractory or relapsed Ta-1 with concomitant Tis or Tis alone, or BCG refractory or relapsed high-grade Ta-1	Intravesical
INSTILADRIN (rAd-IFN/Syn3) (NCT01687244)	Adjuvant	BCG-refractory or relapsed high-grade Ta-1, concomitant Tis, or Tis alone	Intravesical
SCH 72105 with Syn3 (rAd-IFN) (NCT01162785)	Adjuvant	BCG failure X2 or intolerant, recurrent Ta, T1, or Tis	Intravesical

	Setting	Population	Route
Vaccine-based Therapy			
ALT-803 (NCT02138734)	Adjuvant	BCG-naïve, high-risk (high-grade Ta or T1, Tis) or intermediate-risk (recurrent low-grade Ta-1 or low-grade multifocal Ta-1)	Intravesical
ALT-801 (NCT01625260)	Adjuvant	BCG failure or intolerant, high-risk (high-grade Ta-1 or Tis)	Intravesical
recMAGE-A3 + AS15 ASCI (NCT01498172)	Adjuvant	NMIBC	Intramuscular
HS-410 (NCT02010203)	Adjuvant	High risk (high-grade T1, Tis) or intermediate risk (recurrent low-grade Ta or low-grade multifocal Ta)	Subcutaneous
PANVAC (NCT02015104)	Adjuvant	BCG failure, high-grade Ta, T1, and/or Tis	Subcutaneous
Cytotoxic Therapy			
Apaziquone (NCT00598806)	Within 6 h after TURBT	Ta, G1-2	Intravesical
Apaziquone (NCT01410565)	Immediately following TURBT and adjuvant	Multifocal low-grade Ta, or single high-grade Ta	Intravesical
Pembrolizumab (NCT02324582)	Adjuvant	High-grade Ta, T1, and/or Tis	Intravenous
Targeted Therapy			
Tamoxifen (NCT02197897)	Adjuvant	Low- to intermediate-risk NMIBC	Oral
Immune Modulators			
MK-3475 (NCT02324582)	Adjuvant	High-grade Ta, T1, or Tis	Intravenous
Lenalidomide (NCT01373294)	Adjuvant	High-grade Ta, T1, or Tis	Oral
TMX-101 (NCT01731652)	Adjuvant	Tis with or without Ta, T1	Intravesical

and recruitment of myeloid cells as well as functions as a direct inducer of local antitumor immunity. The targeted antitumor activity of CG0070 is finally achieved through preferential replication within RB-defective bladder cancer cells. A phase 1/2 clinical trial treating 35 patients with either single or multiple intravesical treatments and testing several different doses of CG0070 was conducted.[24] Results showed that urinary CG0070 genome levels were found to be markedly elevated above baseline in approximately 90% of the patients. The drug was well tolerated with minimal adverse effects reported. Although not designed to evaluate efficacy, a complete response rate of 48.6% was noted at 10.4 months. An efficacy study for patients with high-grade non-muscle invasive bladder cancer who have received at least 2 prior courses of intravesical therapy is underway (NCT01438112).[19]

Instiladrin

Although interferon-α2b is known to be an important mediator of antitumor immunity, it has not been adequately tested to determine its value as monotherapy for NMIBC. One potential explanation for its limited antitumor capacity is the limited urothelium exposure duration. A recombinant adenovirus-mediated interferon-α2b protein (rAD-IFN-α) attached to SCH 209702 (Syn3) was developed for intravesical therapy of bladder cancer.[25–27] Syn3 is a novel excipient that markedly improves the rate at which adenoviral-mediated transduction of urothelium and NMIBC occurs.[27,28] In a phase 1 trial involving 17 patients, adverse effects were minimal, and the drug was well tolerated; 43% (6 of 13) of patients treated with detectable urine IFN-α levels achieved a complete response at 3 months, with average duration of response lasting 31 months.[29] Of note, 2 patients were disease-free at 29 and 39.2 months. On the other hand, 0% (0 of 1) of patients treated at the same dose, without detectable urine IFN-α levels, achieved complete response. These promising results have led to a phase 2 study for patients with high-grade BCG-refractory or relapsed NMIBC where relapse is defined as recurrence within 1 year after a complete response to BCG treatment (NCT01687244).[19]

BC-819

BC-819 (DTA-H19) is a double-stranded DNA plasmid carrying the gene for the A subunit of diphtheria toxin under the regulation of the H19 gene promoter. H19 is an oncofetal gene encoding for an RNA that acts as a riboregulator and is expressed at high levels in various malignant tissues. A marker lesion study of intravesical BC-819 demonstrated safety and complete ablation of a marker tumor without any new tumor formation in 4 of 18 patients (22% complete response rate).[30] A follow-up study to include 47 patients with intermediate-risk, recurrent, multiple nonmuscle invasive tumors observed complete tumor ablation in 33% of patients and prevented the growth of new tumors in 64% of patients.[31]

Bacillus Calmette-Guérin Modification

In addition to the cytokine-based approach discussed previously, it has been proposed that the primary antineoplastic response of BCG is derived from critical BCG subcomponents of the organism. Several of these subcomponents have also been deemed powerful enough inducers of the Th1 response that they could function as a substitute for live BCG, most notably BCG cell wall skeleton (BCG-CWS) and mycobacterial cell wall component (MCC). If effective, these agents offer the possibility of decreased toxicity and improved adherence to maintenance therapy. Cell wall skeleton derived from Mycobacterium bovis BCG consists of mycolic acid, a long branched chain-hydroxyl fatty acid, and arabinogalactan, a large branch chain heteroglycan. Safety and antitumor activity of cell wall skeleton in patients with bladder cancer awaits clinical evaluation. A mycobacterial cell wall extract prepared from Mycobacterium phlei, an organism that is not pathogenic for people, was tested in patients with CIS and demonstrated tolerability and potential for antitumor activity.[32] It is unclear if such therapies will reach clinical trial testing, as a recent phase 3 trial evaluating the mycobacterial cell wall-DNA complex (EN3348) was terminated due to lack of recruitment (NCT1200992).

Genetic recombination involves bringing together genetic material from different sources, thereby creating novel DNA sequences in biologic organisms. BCG is an effective delivery vehicle for foreign antigens. It has been used as recombinant BCG as a vaccine for human immunodeficiency virus, Mycobacterium tuberculosis, and hepatitis viruses in addition to delivery of tumor-associated antigens such as prostate-specific membrane antigen.[33] BCG's clinical activity is thought to depend in part on eliciting a Th1 immune response characterized by increases in proinflammatory cytokines such as interleukin (IL)-2, INF-γ, IFN-α, and IL-18. Several strains of recombinant BCG have been developed to enhance BCG-induced immune responses by increasing Th1 cytokine production, and clinical investigation of these agents is anticipated.

Vaccine-Based Therapy

There are several vaccine-based therapies that are currently in clinical trials as well. ALT-803 is a recombinant mammalian fusion protein that demonstrates enhanced IL-15 biological activity; it is responsible for proliferation and activation of natural killer cells and CD8[+] memory T cells. A phase 1b/2 study is recruiting high-risk Ta, T1, and CIS patients with BCG intolerance or failure (refractory or relapsing) of at least 1 prior BCG treatment (NCT02138734).[19] ALT-801 is a p53-(T-cell-receptor)-IL-2 fusion protein designed to target cancer cells that overexpress p53, found to occur at high frequency in bladder cancer. This drug is being tested in a phase 1b/2 trial in combination with gemcitabine for patients with BCG failure (NCT01625260).

MAGE-A3 is a potential target for immunotherapy, because it is generally tumor-specific and expressed in many tumor types. A recombinant MAGE-A3 protein (recMAGE-A3), in combination with immunostimulants, induced a significant antigen-specific immune response and eliminated MAGE-A3 expressing tumors in an animal model.[34] A phase 1 clinical trial is underway using recMAGE-A3 in combination with an immunostimulant for patients with NMIBC (NCT01498172).

HS-410 was designed based on various antigens shared among a high proportion of patients with bladder cancer. This therapy claims to use bladder cancer cells to stimulate the patient's immune system to activate immune responses against a range of antigens including bladder cancer-specific antigens. Details on the construct are lacking on the specific nature of these proteins. A phase 1/2 placebo-controlled trial is currently underway for patients with intermediate and high-risk NMIBC (NCT02010203).

carcinoembryonic antigen (CEA) and MUC-1 are overexpressed in a large number of solid tumors, and vaccines directed against these proteins can facilitate immune responses against tumors harboring these proteins. Ideally, by stimulating immune responses, tumor vaccines could facilitate breaking of immunologic tolerance toward tumors generally, not necessarily tumors harboring these specific proteins. PANVAC [poxviral vaccine regimen with genes for CEA and MUC-1 along with TRICOM (B7.1, ICAM-1 and LFA-3)] is a poxviral vaccine regimen consisting of genes for CEA and MUC-1, along with a triad of costimulatory molecules (TRICOM; composed of B7.1, intercellular adhesion molecule 1, and lymphocyte function-associated antigen 3) engineered into vaccinia (PANVAC-V) as a prime vaccination, and into fowlpox (PANVAC-F) as a booster vaccination. A trial is currently underway and aims to enroll patients with high-grade Ta, T1 and CIS bladder cancer (NCT02015104).[19]

Cytotoxic Agents

Apaziquone

Apaziquone, (EO9), is a synthetic indoloquinone-based bioreductive alkylating agent that becomes cytotoxic following activation by the enzyme deoxythymidine–diaphorase. Deoxythymidine–diaphorase is preferentially expressed at higher concentrations within bladder cancer cells, leading to the potential for targeted anticancer therapy. Because of this, apaziquone was demonstrated as needing 6 to 78 times less concentration than that of MMC to achieve 50% cell death, depending upon the bladder cancer cell line utilized. A marker lesion study demonstrated a complete response in 67.4% of 46 patients with Ta-T1 G1-2 bladder cancer.[35] In a phase 2 study of intermediate- and high-risk patients, recurrent tumors were seen in only 34.7% of patients at 1 year, and only 1 patient had progressed to muscle-invasive disease.[36] These results prompted phase 3 trials of single-dose intravesical apaziquone (EOquin) in the early postoperative period for patients undergoing transurethral resection of NMIBC (NCT00598806) and multiple instillations as adjuvant therapy (NCT01410565).

Pirarubicin

Pirarubicin, an anthracycline analogue of doxorubicin, functions via 2 different mechanisms. It directly inhibits DNA replication and repair through DNA intercalation, and it interacts with topoisomerase II, thereby preventing adequate RNA and protein synthesis.[37] A clinical study of single post-TURBT instillation of pirarubicin in patients with Ta-T1 bladder cancer demonstrated nonrecurrence rates of 92.4%, 82.7%, and 78.8% at 1, 2, and 3-year follow-up, respectively.[38] In addition, a randomized study of Ta-T1 bladder cancer subjected to post-TURBT pirarubicin and weekly treatment for 8 weeks versus 8 weekly treatments demonstrated recurrence rates of 7.8% and 14.3% at 18-month follow-up, respectively.[39]

Targeted Therapies

Oportuzumab monatox

Epithelial cell adhesion molecule (EpCAM) overexpression has been associated with higher grade of bladder cancer. Oportuzumab monatox (OM) is a recombinant fusion protein of humanized anti-EpCAM antibody linked to *Pseudomonas* exotoxin A. Once OM is bound to the bladder cancer cell in question and internalized, the exotoxin induces apoptosis. A phase 2 trial involving 45 total patients evaluated 2 OM dosing strategies, specifically focusing on BCG-refractory carcinoma in situ.[40] Both treatment schedules were based upon a prior study using OM, with an initial induction cycle followed by 3 weekly instillations at 3-month intervals. OM demonstrated complete response rates of 26.7% and 15.6% at the 6- and 12-month intervals, respectively.

Tamoxifen

Tamoxifen belongs to the class of medications known as selective estrogen receptor modulators, which function as agonists of estrogen receptors in certain tissues (endometrium) and antagonists in others (breast). Although it is widely known that bladder cancer has a much higher prevalence in men, several studies have theorized this is because of increased estrogen levels in women. For example, late menopause and use of oral contraceptives and hormone replacement therapy are associated with lower risk of bladder cancer.[41] Estrogen receptors (ERs) have been demonstrated to be expressed in normal urothelium as well as bladder cancer, with ERβ detected in up to 81% of bladder cancers; increased levels of expression are associated with higher-grade tumors.[42] Preclinical evidence for antiproliferation of bladder tumors with tamoxifen has been observed. Female mice were given a known bladder-specific carcinogen, N-butyl-N-(4-hydroxylbutyl) nitrosamine (BBN), which resulted in 76% tumor incidence in the control group and only 10% to 14% incidence in the tamoxifen-treated group.[43] Tamoxifen is currently being evaluated in a phase 2 study of low- to intermediate-risk NMIBC, with a focus on pharmacodynamic effects (NCT02197897).[19]

Immune Modulators

Checkpoint inhibitors

Novel checkpoint inhibitors, including PD-1 and PD-L1 inhibitors, have demonstrated impressive and durable antitumor response in advanced, metastatic bladder cancer, and this has prompted considerations for testing in NMIBC. Currently there is one trial utilizing a checkpoint inhibitor in combination with BCG listed in clinicaltrials.gov, but others are expected. The PD-1 inhibitor, pembrolizumab (also known as MK-3475), is being tested in a phase 1 study in combination with BCG for patients with high-risk NMIBC (NCT02324582).

Lenalidomide

Lenalidomide, an analogue of thalidomide, has several known mechanisms of action and is currently FDA approved for the treatment of specific types of myelodysplastic syndrome and multiple myeloma. It inhibits angiogenesis, induces tumor cell apoptosis, and has an immunomodulatory role. In a preclinical trial, lenalidomide, in combination with BCG, was evaluated for its efficacy in MBT-2 cell lines implanted in immunocompetent mice, with results demonstrating a statistically significant decrease in tumor size.[44] Lenalidomide is being tested in combination with BCG in a phase 2 trial of high-risk NMIBC (NCT01373294).[19]

Toll-like receptor agonist

Toll-like receptors (TLRs) are pattern-recognition receptors, which, when activated, alert the immune system to presence of microbes and are primary signaling mechanisms for the innate immune response. TLR agonists are a promising target for bladder cancer therapy, as BCG is a known TLR agonist. Imiquimod is a TLR-7 agonist and is FDA approved for the treatment of superficial basal cell carcinoma. TLR-7 agonists have been tested in preclinical models of bladder cancer, with some evidence of antitumor activity.[45,46] In the clinical setting, TMX-101, a variant formulation of imiquimod, was tested in a phase 1 trial demonstrating safety in 16 patients.[47] A phase 2 trial (NCT01731652) has been developed.[19]

SUMMARY AND FUTURE DIRECTIONS

BCG immunotherapy remains the mainstay of therapy for NMIBC since its initial use several decades ago. Novel therapies in bladder cancer will likely benefit from the remarkable clinical activity of BCG and include strategies such as recombinant or subcomponent BCG. Delivery of therapy into the bladder is an exciting area of research, with several agents showing promise in early studies. It is anticipated that the future approach to treating NMIBC will be impacted, to some extent, by emerging novel immunotherapies, and strategic clinical trials will be required for rapid translation of these new modalities into clinical practice.

REFERENCES

1. Siegel R, Ma J, Zou Z, et al. Cancer statistics, 2014. CA Cancer J Clin 2014;64:9–29.
2. Zlotta AR, Fleshner NE, Jewett MA. The management of BCG failure in non-muscle-invasive bladder cancer: an update. Can Urol Assoc J 2009;3:S199–205.
3. GuhaSarkar S, Banerjee R. Intravesical drug delivery: challenges, current status, opportunities and novel strategies. J Control Release 2010;148:147–59.
4. Wientjes MG, Badalament RA, Wang RC, et al. Penetration of mitomycin C in human bladder. Cancer Res 1993;53:3314–20.

5. Di Stasi SM, Vespasiani G, Giannantoni A, et al. Electromotive delivery of mitomycin C into human bladder wall. Cancer Res 1997;57:875–80.

6. Di Stasi SM, Giannantoni A, Giurioli A, et al. Sequential BCG and electromotive mitomycin versus BCG alone for high-risk superficial bladder cancer: a randomised controlled trial. Lancet Oncol 2006;7:43–51.

7. Di Stasi SM, Valenti M, Verri C, et al. Electromotive instillation of mitomycin immediately before transurethral resection for patients with primary urothelial non-muscle invasive bladder cancer: a randomised controlled trial. Lancet Oncol 2011;12:871–9.

8. Sparreboom A, Scripture CD, Trieu V, et al. Comparative preclinical and clinical pharmacokinetics of a cremophor-free, nanoparticle albumin-bound paclitaxel (ABI-007) and paclitaxel formulated in Cremophor (Taxol). Clin Cancer Res 2005;11:4136–43.

9. McKiernan JM, Barlow LJ, Laudano MA, et al. A phase I trial of intravesical nanoparticle albumin-bound paclitaxel in the treatment of bacillus Calmette-Guerin refractory nonmuscle invasive bladder cancer. J Urol 2011;186:448–51.

10. McKiernan JM, Holder DD, Ghandour RA, et al. Phase II trial of intravesical nanoparticle albumin bound paclitaxel for the treatment of nonmuscle invasive urothelial carcinoma of the bladder after bacillus Calmette-Guerin treatment failure. J Urol 2014;192:1633–8.

11. Jagannath C, Lindsey DR, Dhandayuthapani S, et al. Autophagy enhances the efficacy of BCG vaccine by increasing peptide presentation in mouse dendritic cells. Nat Med 2009;15:267–76.

12. Seager CM, Puzio-Kuter AM, Patel T, et al. Intravesical delivery of rapamycin suppresses tumorigenesis in a mouse model of progressive bladder cancer. Cancer Prev Res (Phila) 2009;2:1008–14.

13. Niranjan R, Koushik C, Saravanan S, et al. A novel injectable temperature-sensitive zinc doped chitosan/beta-glycerophosphate hydrogel for bone tissue engineering. Int J Biol Macromol 2013;54:24–9.

14. Delto JC, Kobayashi T, Benson M, et al. Preclinical analyses of intravesical chemotherapy for prevention of bladder cancer progression. Oncotarget 2013;4:269–76.

15. Arends TJ, van der Heijden AG, Witjes JA. Combined chemohyperthermia: 10-year single center experience in 160 patients with nonmuscle invasive bladder cancer. J Urol 2014;192:708–13.

16. Colombo R, Salonia A, Leib Z, et al. Long-term outcomes of a randomized controlled trial comparing thermochemotherapy with mitomycin-C alone as adjuvant treatment for non-muscle-invasive bladder cancer (NMIBC). BJU Int 2011;107:912–8.

17. Kiss B, Schneider S, Thalmann GN, et al. Is thermochemotherapy with the Synergo system a viable treatment option in patients with recurrent non-muscle-invasive bladder cancer? Int J Urol 2014; 22(2):158–62.

18. Inman BA, Stauffer PR, Craciunescu OA, et al. A pilot clinical trial of intravesical mitomycin-C and external deep pelvic hyperthermia for non-muscle-invasive bladder cancer. Int J Hyperthermia 2014; 30:171–5.

19. NIH. vol. 2015. Available at: ClinicalTrials.gov. 2014. Accessed January 3, 2015.

20. Loskog A, Dzojic H, Vikman S, et al. Adenovirus CD40 ligand gene therapy counteracts immune escape mechanisms in the tumor Microenvironment. J Immunol 2004;172:7200–5.

21. Malmstrom PU, Loskog AS, Lindqvist CA, et al. AdCD40L immunogene therapy for bladder carcinoma–the first phase I/IIa trial. Clin Cancer Res 2010;16:3279–87.

22. Miyamoto H, Shuin T, Torigoe S, Iwasaki Y, Kubota Y. Retinoblastoma gene mutations in primary human bladder cancer. British J Cancer 1995;71:831–5.

23. Ramesh N, Ge Y, Ennist DL, et al. CG0070, a conditionally replicating granulocyte macrophage colony-stimulating factor–armed oncolytic adenovirus for the treatment of bladder cancer. Clin Cancer Res 2006;12:305–13.

24. Burke JM, Lamm DL, Meng MV, et al. A first in human phase 1 study of CG0070, a GM-CSF expressing oncolytic adenovirus, for the treatment of nonmuscle invasive bladder cancer. J Urol 2012; 188:2391–7.

25. Nagabhushan TL, Maneval DC, Benedict WF, et al. Enhancement of intravesical delivery with Syn3 potentiates interferon-alpha2b gene therapy for superficial bladder cancer. Cytokine Growth Factor Rev 2007;18:389–94.

26. Tao Z, Connor RJ, Ashoori F, et al. Efficacy of a single intravesical treatment with Ad-IFN/Syn 3 is dependent on dose and urine IFN concentration obtained: implications for clinical investigation. Cancer Gene Ther 2006;13:125–30.

27. Benedict WF, Tao Z, Kim CS, et al. Intravesical Ad-IFNalpha causes marked regression of human bladder cancer growing orthotopically in nude mice and overcomes resistance to IFN-alpha protein. Mol Ther 2004;10:525–32.

28. Connor RJ, Anderson JM, Machemer T, et al. Sustained intravesical interferon protein exposure is achieved using an adenoviral-mediated gene delivery system: a study in rats evaluating dosing regimens. Urology 2005;66:224–9.

29. Dinney CP, Fisher MB, Navai N, et al. Phase I trial of intravesical recombinant adenovirus mediated interferon-alpha2b formulated in Syn3 for Bacillus Calmette-Guerin failures in nonmuscle invasive bladder cancer. J Urol 2013;190:850–6.

30. Sidi AA, Ohana P, Benjamin S, et al. Phase I/II marker lesion study of intravesical BC-819 DNA plasmid in H19 over expressing superficial bladder

cancer refractory to bacillus Calmette-Guerin. J Urol 2008;180:2379–83.

31. Gofrit ON, Benjamin S, Halachmi S, et al. DNA based therapy with diphtheria toxin-A BC-819: a phase 2b marker lesion trial in patients with intermediate risk nonmuscle invasive bladder cancer. J Urol 2014;191:1697–702.

32. Morales A, Chin JL, Ramsey EW. Mycobacterial cell wall extract for treatment of carcinoma in situ of the bladder. J Urol 2001;166:1633–7 [discussion: 1637–8].

33. Luo Y, Henning J, O'Donnell MA. Th1 cytokine-secreting recombinant Mycobacterium bovis bacillus Calmette-Guerin and prospective use in immunotherapy of bladder cancer. Clin Dev Immunol 2011;2011:728930.

34. Gerard C, Baudson N, Ory T, et al. Tumor mouse model confirms MAGE-A3 cancer immunotherapeutic as an efficient inducer of long-lasting antitumoral responses. PLoS One 2014;9:e94883.

35. Hendricksen K, van der Heijden AG, Cornel EB, et al. Two-year follow-up of the phase II marker lesion study of intravesical apaziquone for patients with non-muscle invasive bladder cancer. World J Urol 2009;27:337–42.

36. Hendricksen K, Cornel EB, de Reijke TM, et al. Phase 2 study of adjuvant intravesical instillations of apaziquone for high risk nonmuscle invasive bladder cancer. J Urol 2012;187:1195–9.

37. Li Q, Xu T, Wang XF. Mechanism of intravesical instillation of pirarubicin for preventing recurrence of non-muscle invasive bladder cancer. Zhonghua zhong liu za zhi 2009;31:904–7 [in Chinese].

38. Okamura K, Ono Y, Kinukawa T, et al. Randomized study of single early instillation of (2″R)-4'-O-tetrahydropyranyl-doxorubicin for a single superficial bladder carcinoma. Cancer 2002;94:2363–8.

39. Li NC, Ye ZQ, Na YQ, CUA THP Immediate Instillations Study Group. Efficacy of immediate instillation combined with regular instillations of pirarubicin for Ta and T1 transitional cell bladder cancer after transurethral resection: a prospective, randomized, multicenter study. Chin Med J 2013;126:2805–9.

40. Kowalski M, Guindon J, Brazas L, et al. A phase II study of oportuzumab monatox: an immunotoxin therapy for patients with noninvasive urothelial carcinoma in situ previously treated with bacillus Calmette-Guerin. J Urol 2012;188:1712–8.

41. McGrath M, Michaud DS, De Vivo I. Hormonal and reproductive factors and the risk of bladder cancer in women. Am J Epidemiol 2006;163:236–44.

42. Abstracts of papers presented at the thirtieth annual meeting of the American Society for Cell Biology. San Diego, California. December 9–13, 1990. The Journal of Cell Biology 111, 1a-511a (1990).

43. George SK, Tovar-Sepulveda V, Shen SS, et al. Chemoprevention of BBN-induced bladder carcinogenesis by the selective estrogen receptor modulator tamoxifen. Transl Oncol 2013;6:244–55.

44. Jinesh GG, Lee EK, Tran J, et al. Lenalidomide augments the efficacy of bacillus Calmette-Guerin (BCG) immunotherapy in vivo. Urol Oncol 2013;31:1676–82.

45. Smith EB, Schwartz M, Kawamoto H, et al. Antitumor effects of imidazoquinolines in urothelial cell carcinoma of the bladder. J Urol 2007;177:2347–51.

46. Hayashi T, Crain B, Corr M, et al. Intravesical toll-like receptor 7 agonist R-837: optimization of its formulation in an orthotopic mouse model of bladder cancer. Int J Urol 2010;17:483–90.

47. Falke J, Lammers RJ, Arentsen HC, et al. Results of a phase 1 dose escalation study of intravesical TMX-101 in patients with nonmuscle invasive bladder cancer. J Urol 2013;189:2077–82.

Trimodality Therapy in Bladder Cancer
Who, What, and When?

Christopher Premo, MD[a], Andrea B. Apolo, MD[b],
Piyush K. Agarwal, MD[c], Deborah E. Citrin, MD[a,*]

KEYWORDS

- Radiation • Bladder preservation • Muscle-invasive bladder cancer • Chemoradiation
- Urothelial carcinoma of the bladder

KEY POINTS

- Bladder preservation with maximal transurethral resection of the bladder tumor (TURBT), concurrent chemotherapy, and irradiation can result in approximately 75% of long-term survivors maintaining a functional bladder.
- The ideal patient for bladder preservation has a clinical T2 unifocal tumor, a visibly complete TURBT, no carcinoma in situ (CIS), and no tumor-related hydronephrosis, with good pretreatment bladder function.
- Participation in a bladder preservation approach requires a highly motivated patient who is a good candidate for irradiation and chemotherapy and is committed to long-term cystoscopic surveillance.

INTRODUCTION

An estimated 74,690 cases of urinary bladder cancer were diagnosed in the United States in 2014,[1] of which 30% will be muscle invasive. The current standard of care for the treatment of muscle-invasive bladder cancer (MIBC) is neoadjuvant cisplatin-based chemotherapy followed by radical cystectomy (RC) with pelvic lymph node dissection.[2] In appropriately selected patients, bladder preservation can be an effective alternative to RC. The term bladder preservation can include TURBT, limited surgery, chemotherapy, radiation therapy, or various combinations of one or more

of these modalities; however, the best outcomes have consistently been seen with trimodality therapy (TMT) including maximal TURBT followed by concurrent chemoradiation. This review focuses on TMT for bladder preservation and does not detail other therapeutic combinations for bladder preservation.

Several prospective trials have been completed evaluating TMT as a means of bladder preservation. The purpose of these studies has been to define the rate of bladder preservation and survival with this approach and to improve the tolerability and efficacy of TMT regimens. This review

This research was supported by the Intramural Research Program of the National Institutes of Health, National Cancer Institute.

Disclosures and conflicts of interests: The authors have no conflicts of interests or relationships to disclose.

[a] Radiation Oncology Branch, Center for Cancer Research, National Cancer Institute, 10 CRC, B2-3500, Bethesda, MD 20892, USA; [b] Bladder Cancer Section, Genitourinary Malignancies Branch, Center for Cancer Research, National Cancer Institute, National Institutes of Health, 10 Center Drive 12N226, MSC 1906, Bethesda, MD 20892, USA; [c] Bladder Cancer Section, Urologic Oncology Branch, National Cancer Institute, National Institutes of Health, Building 10, Room 2W-5940, Bethesda, MD 20892-1210, USA

* Corresponding author.

E-mail address: citrind@mail.nih.gov

provides an overview of modern TMT bladder-preservation strategies, focusing on important criteria for patient selection, the integration of novel radiation techniques, commonly used and new chemotherapies for TMT, and the role of chemoradiation for T1 disease.

DISCUSSION
Trimodality Therapy Treatment Approach

TMT includes the combination of maximal tumor debulking and concurrent chemoradiotherapy. The optimal radiation target volume, radiation fractionation, chemotherapy, and sequencing remain areas of active study. In general, the patient undergoes a maximal, preferably visually complete, TURBT, ideally with bladder mapping (**Fig. 1**), followed by the delivery of cisplatin-based chemoradiotherapy to a dose of approximately 40 to 45 Gy. If no evidence of disease or minimal residual disease is noted at cystoscopic reassessment, the final consolidative phase of chemoradiotherapy is initiated. If progressive or unresponsive disease is found, therapy proceeds to RC. After completion of therapy, patients are closely surveilled with cystoscopy and urine cytology.

Patient Selection

Patient selection is a key component of bladder preservation (**Table 1**). Most criteria used to select appropriate patients for TMT predict for a high rate of response or the ability to safely tolerate therapy. Factors predicting for increased rates of distant metastases are important for predicting overall survival (OS) after TMT.

A complete response (CR) to induction therapy with concurrent chemoradiation has typically been defined as negative results on urine cytologic analysis, as well as no visible tumor and negative results on biopsies at cystoscopy. Achieving a CR to induction therapy is required to avoid salvage cystectomy and has been associated with improved disease-free and overall survival after TMT. The CR rate for patients with T2-T4a disease treated with TMT is approximately 70%.[3] Factors that may affect the likelihood of achieving a CR after TMT and should be considered when selecting patients include completeness of TURBT, tumor stage, hydronephrosis, multifocality and CIS, and baseline bladder function. It is important to consider that the rate of response to induction therapy may not always be known, as many recent trials, such as bladder cancer 2001 (BC2001) and Radiation Therapy Oncology Group (RTOG) 0926, do not include cystoscopic reassessment after induction. For these studies, careful patient selection becomes increasingly important as a full

radiotherapy (RT) dose is delivered before response to therapy is assessed.

Completeness of transurethral resection of the bladder tumor

A pooled analysis of 314 patients treated on 6 RTOG trials found that a visibly complete TURBT was associated with a significantly higher rate of CR to TMT on multivariate analaysis.[3] Similarly, the Erlangen series showed that completeness of resection after initial TURBT was an independent predictor of CR.[4] Likewise, a series of 348 patients from Massachusetts General Hospital found that visibly complete TURBT was associated with higher CR rates (79% with visibly complete TURBT vs 57% without).[5] Thus, a visibly complete TURBT is ideal. A less-than-complete TURBT is not an absolute contraindication to bladder preservation, as several trials have demonstrated acceptable CR rates without a visibly complete TURBT.

Tumor stage

Most TMT trials include patients with clinical T2-T4a disease. In RTOG 85-12, RTOG 88-02, RTOG 97-06, and the Erlangen series, tumor stage was not significantly associated with the rate of CR to TMT on multivariate analysis.[4,6–8] A pooled analysis of 361 patients treated on RTOG trials confirmed that T stage did not predict for the likelihood of CR to TMT on multivariate analysis.[3] In contrast, increasing T stage is reproducibly associated with reduced long-term survival after TMT.[4,5,9]

In surgical series, the presence of prostate invasion by urothelial carcinoma is associated with a higher risk of lymph node metastases and reduced 5-year survival.[10] The decrement in survival is greatest for patients with prostatic stromal invasion or extraprostatic invasion compared with patients with more limited mucosal involvement. Patients with prostatic stromal invasion are excluded from many trials of TMT for bladder preservation; however, prostatic urethral invasion is not generally an exclusion criterion if it is amenable to visibly complete resection.

Few data exist regarding the treatment of patients with involved lymph nodes with TMT. These patients have in some cases been included in RTOG trials of TMT if the lymph nodes are located below the bifurcation of the iliac vessels. The presence of lymph node involvement is a poor prognostic indicator in regards to OS, and in general, these patients are counseled to undergo neoadjuvant chemotherapy and RC.

Hydronephrosis

Tumor-related hydronephrosis has been an exclusion criterion for several trials of TMT. RTOG 89-03

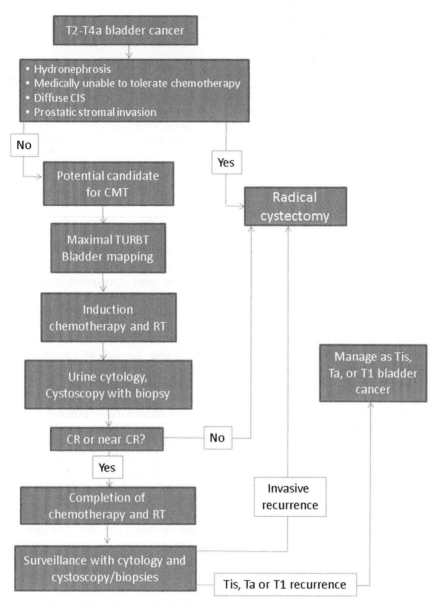

Fig. 1. Sequencing of trimodality therapy for bladder preservation. Patients undergoing TMT for bladder preservation undergo a maximal TURBT followed by induction chemoradiation. Patients with a CR to induction therapy proceed to consolidative chemoradiation, whereas evidence of progression results in immediate cystectomy. Following therapy, a strict schedule of surveillance is undertaken. Evidence of invasive recurrence is treated with cystectomy. Noninvasive recurrences are managed with TURBT and intravesicle therapy.

found CR rates with and without hydronephrosis to be 38% and 64%, respectively. A series from the Massachusetts General Hospital found a CR rate of 52% in those with hydronephrosis and 77% in those without.[11] Hydronephrosis not only predicts for a reduced likelihood of CR but also is a predictor for advanced stage and decreased survival. In RTOG 89-03, the 5-year OS for patients with and without hydronephrosis was 33% and 54%, respectively.[12] Likewise, in RTOG 88-02, hydronephrosis was the only analyzed factor to be significantly associated with probability of distant metastases and death.[7] Patients with tumor-related hydronephrosis are poor candidates for bladder preservation and are usually excluded from trials of TMT.

Multifocality and carcinoma in situ

Multiple tumors or multifocal disease has been suggested as a predictive factor for decreased response rates to TMT, and patients with these conditions are excluded from most trials of

Table 1
Patient selection for bladder preservation

Preferred or Ideal	Less than Ideal	Relative Contraindications	Absolute Contraindications
T2	T3a	T3b-T4a	T4b
No hydronephrosis	Incomplete TURBT	Diffuse CIS	Tumor-Related Hydronephrosis
No CIS	Multifocal tumor	Lymph node positive disease	Prior pelvic radiation therapy
Visibly complete TURBT	Poor bladder function or capacity		Not a candidate for chemotherapy
Unifocal tumor			Prostatic stromal invasion
Good bladder function and capacity			

bladder preservation. Multifocality may not predict for lower rates of CR but is associated with a higher risk for local relapse.[4] In general, TMT is not advocated in those with diffuse multifocal disease.

Similarly, the presence of extensive CIS before therapy has been associated with lower rates of CR to TMT and RT alone and higher rates of recurrence after TMT.[13–16] A panel convened by the Société Internationale d'Urologie suggested that the presence of extensive CIS should be considered a relative and not absolute contraindication to TMT because the presence of CIS affects only the risk of recurrence after TMT and not survival.[17]

Baseline bladder function

The rationale of bladder preservation therapy is to preserve a functional bladder. A subset of patients whose bladders are preserved with TMT may develop symptoms such as urgency and control problems.[18] Therefore, baseline dysfunction in these areas should be considered when determining if a patient is a candidate for TMT.

Chemotherapy for Trimodality Therapy

Concurrent chemotherapy has been shown in randomized trials to improve local and regional control compared with RT alone.[19,20] Although these trials did not demonstrate an OS advantage with the addition of concurrent chemotherapy, several large retrospective series have found concurrent chemotherapy to be associated with improved survival.[9,21] Most bladder preservation trials using concurrent chemoradiation have used cisplatin-based chemotherapy regimens. Cisplatin-based combination regimens have been tested with the aim of improving response rates. The RTOG has evaluated cisplatin-based chemotherapy combinations including cisplatin with 5-fluorouracil (5-FU) (RTOG 9506) and paclitaxel with

cisplatin (RTOG 9906).[22,23] The RTOG 0233 trial compared paclitaxel with cisplatin with 5-FU with cisplatin with concurrent radiation in patients with mostly T2 disease (95%).[24] Following TMT, patients received adjuvant gemcitabine, cisplatin, and paclitaxel. Both regimens showed similar rates of CR (62%–72%), 5-year OS (71%–75%), and 5-year survival with an intact bladder with moderate toxicity.

Candidates for TMT may have comorbidities that preclude the delivery of concurrent cisplatin, and several studies have evaluated alternative regimens. The BC2001 trial tested the use of 5-FU with mitomycin-C (MMC) concurrently with RT with excellent response rates and impressive tolerability.[19] This regimen is particularly useful in those with renal dysfunction prohibiting the use of cisplatin. Gemcitabine is a potent radiation sensitizer and has shown activity in the setting of metastatic urothelial cancers. The use of 100 mg/m^2 weekly gemcitabine during RT as a component of TMT was tested in a recently completed phase II trial.[25] The regimen resulted in an 88% cystoscopic response rate and a 3-year OS of 75%. Bowel toxicity resulted in 4 of 50 patients stopping chemotherapy and in 1 late bowel resection. There were 2 treatment-related deaths.

Single-institution phase I data supporting twice-weekly gemcitabine concurrent with RT as part of TMT are available. A study from the University of Michigan of TMT with RT delivered to a total dose of 60 Gy found the maximum tolerated dose of twice-weekly gemcitabine to be 27 mg/m^2.[26] Of the 23 patients treated in this trial, 21 obtained a CR. At a median follow-up of 43 months, 65% of patients were alive with no evidence of recurrence and intact bladders. Twice-weekly low-dose gemcitabine (27 mg/m^2) was compared with a regimen of twice-daily irradiation with 5-FU and cisplatin in the recently closed RTOG 0712 trial. Results for this trial are pending.

The target volume of radiation is an important consideration when comparing chemotherapy regimens for bladder cancer. Some trials testing alternative regimens have evaluated bladder only irradiation and have not included an initial pelvic irradiation field.[19] Thus, toxicity for these chemotherapy regimens may be greater if extrapolated to a setting in which a pelvic field is included.

The use of neoadjuvant cisplatin-based chemotherapy in the setting of cystectomy has shown improvements in survival compared with cystectomy alone, likely through early treatment of micrometastatic disease.[27,28] As distant failure remains a concern after bladder preservation, this approach has been tested in several trials of TMT. Unfortunately, neoadjuvant or adjuvant chemotherapy with TMT has not improved survival or bladder preservation rates. However, the data available are limited to older regimens, with only 2 cycles of chemotherapy delivered instead of the standard 3 to 4, and many of these studies were underpowered. As more effective chemotherapeutic regimens are developed, this strategy is likely to be further explored.[29]

Targeted agents have been an area of interest in efforts to improve TMT outcomes. The epidermal growth factor receptor family of receptors has been of particular interest in this regard. HER2/Neu is overexpressed in bladder cancers, particularly in metastatic or lymph node–positive tumors,[30] and overexpression may be correlated to worse outcomes after chemoradiotherapy.[31] These findings suggest that targeting HER2/Neu in the context of TMT may provide a therapeutic opportunity. RTOG 0524 evaluated the addition of trastuzumab to paclitaxel and daily irradiation following TURBT in the treatment of noncystectomy candidates with MIBC.[32] The study has been reported as an abstract and showed a favorable response rate but with an increase in hematologic toxicity and other adverse events.

Radiation Techniques

RT is a critical component of TMT. A range of doses of irradiation, fractionation schedules, sequences of treatment, and treatment volumes have been applied in the treatment of bladder cancer. Attempts to improve RT have been geared toward enhancing bladder preservation rates while minimizing the toxicity of therapy. Newer technologies, such as intensity-modulated radiotherapy (IMRT) and image-guided radiotherapy (IGRT), are being integrated into the clinic. The authors outline general concepts regarding RT field design and discuss current areas of research in RT technique.

The optimal volume of irradiation is one area of controversy. In most North American trials, treatment includes an initial course of RT to a total dose of 39.6 to 45 Gy directed at the pelvic lymph nodes below the bifurcation of the common iliac vessels, the prostate in men, and the whole bladder (**Figs. 2** and **3**). A margin surrounding the bladder is included to account for daily variation in bladder filling, visceral organ motion, and setup error. To minimize the field size and to increase the reproducibility of daily treatment, patients are simulated and treated with an empty bladder (immediately postvoid) with a small amount of bladder contrast.

The rationale for including pelvic lymph nodes in the initial portion of the radiation treatment field relates to the high rate of occult lymph node involvement in regions typically targeted with pelvic RT[33] and the finding that extensive lymphadenectomy at the time of RC improves survival, suggesting that treatment of these lymph nodes has therapeutic efficacy.[34] The rationale for not specifically targeting pelvic lymph nodes includes improving tolerability of therapy by excluding more normal tissue from the treatment volume and the low rate of nodal failure when not specifically targeted.

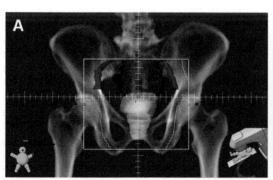
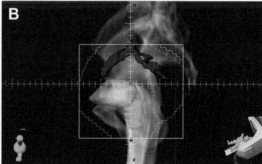

Fig. 2. Pelvic radiation field for bladder preservation. (*A*) Anterior-to-posterior and (*B*) left lateral field. The fields extend from the top of the bifurcation of the iliac vessels to the bottom of the pelvis. The bladder (*yellow*) and prostate (*green*) with margin are included in the target volume. Field edges are noted in yellow.

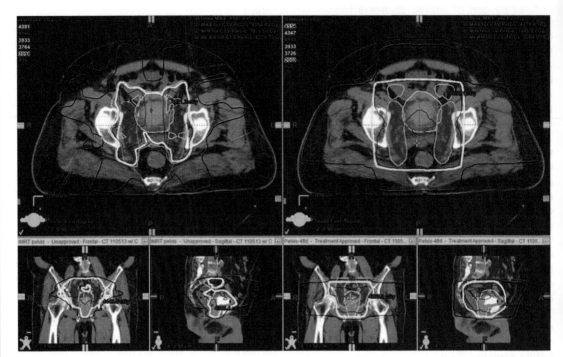

Fig. 3. IMRT for bladder preservation. A comparison of IMRT (*left panels*) and standard 4-field plan (*right panels*) for treatment of the pelvis as a component of bladder preservation. The bladder and prostate (*shaded yellow*) and lower pelvic lymph nodes (*shaded green*) are targeted. Radiation isodose levels are noted in the top left and are represented by the corresponding colored line. Note the superior sparing of the rectum and nontarget tissues with the IMRT approach.

A small, single-institution trial including patients with T2-T4N0 disease treated with maximal TURBT followed by chemoradiation with weekly cisplatin randomized patients between whole-pelvis RT versus bladder-only RT.[35] At a median follow-up of 5 years, no difference in 5-year disease-free survival, bladder preservation rates, regional nodal failure rates, or 5-year OS was observed. In the randomized BC2001 trial comparing irradiation alone with irradiation with chemotherapy, pelvic lymph nodes were not specifically targeted, and pelvic relapses were seen in only 5.8% of patients, suggesting that treatment of the pelvic lymph nodes may not be necessary.[19] Although the authors concluded that bladder-alone RT was as effective as whole-pelvis RT with less toxicity in their trial, a randomized trial comparing these techniques directly is warranted.

If the pelvic lymph nodes are irradiated, 1 or 2 reductions in the size of the fields are performed after the pelvic nodal portion of the treatment. A further area of controversy and ongoing evolution in treatment practices is the volume included in the reduced treatment field, which may include the entire bladder for all or part of the treatment or only the tumor with margin. The rationale for using a tumor-only boost is the ability to reduce the volume of bladder receiving the higher doses of radiation, thus potentially reducing long-term urinary and gastrointestinal toxicity. Although the most common approach is to treat only the residual tumor/tumor bed to the high dose of radiation (~64 Gy) with partial bladder irradiation after delivery of approximately 54 Gy to the whole bladder, this can be challenging for several reasons. For one, after complete TURBT, it can be difficult to know exactly where the pre-TURBT tumor was located despite using the operative report and bladder mapping. In addition, targeting the region accurately can be difficult on a day-to-day basis, as the bladder can have significant interfraction and intrafraction movement due to differences in bladder filling, rectal volume changes, and other variations in organ motion.[36,37] If a tumor bed boost technique is used, accurate tumor delineation and accurate treatment delivery are critical.

Data supporting a more limited boost include the BC2001 trial, in which 219 patients were randomized to receive full-dose radiation to the bladder alone versus 80% of the dose to the bladder with full dose to the bladder tumor/tumor bed.[19] There was no significant difference in toxicity or local control; however, the investigators concluded noninferiority of locoregional control could not be concluded formally. Additional trials have demonstrated comparable control rates with RT directed at the tumor as opposed to the whole bladder, suggesting that this approach does not compromise tumor control.[38,39]

New Radiation Techniques

Recent advances in RT delivery have included the development of IMRT, in which the beam is modulated over the course of the treatment, resulting in improved conformality and a reduction in the amount of normal tissues exposed to higher doses. This technique has been adopted in a wide range of tumor types as a method to improve the conformality of treatment and reduce toxicity, and there have been some reports of the use of IMRT for the treatment of bladder cancer.[40,41] Although a reduction in toxicity that may be afforded by IMRT is welcome, one of the concerns using IMRT is the possibility of marginal misses in regions where there can be considerable organ/target motion. Thus, inclusion of advanced imaging techniques for daily radiation treatment setup is encouraged if IMRT is used.

The ability to accurately define the high-risk region for a whole bladder and partial bladder boost on a daily basis may improve normal tissue sparing by allowing a reduction in the additional margin of normal tissues that must be included to account for setup error. The use of frequent 2-dimensional or 3-dimensional imaging to align patients for daily treatment is known as IGRT. IGRT can be accomplished with daily in-room computed tomographic (CT) scanning (on-board imaging with cone beam CT, **Fig. 4**) or daily imaging of fiducial markers implanted within or near the target volume (see **Fig. 3**). Although fiducial markers have not been widely used in the treatment of bladder cancer, Garcia and colleagues[42] published their experience with fiducial marker placement in the bladder wall for daily localization. In this small series, fiducial marker placement was feasible and associated with excellent retention and no complications. Alternatives to fiducial markers, such as lipiodol injections in the bladder wall, have also been used to assist with accurate daily alignment.[43]

Outcomes of Trimodality Therapy

Although no randomized trials compare RC with bladder preservation in patients with MIBC, many trials, prospective and retrospective, show outcomes similar to those obtained after RC in regards to OS (**Table 2**). Following maximal TURBT, definitive treatment with concurrent chemoradiation

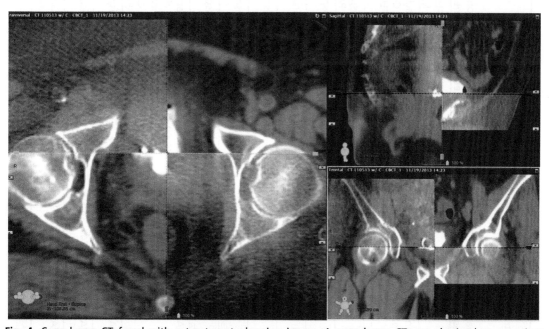

Fig. 4. Cone beam CT fused with a treatment planning image. A cone beam CT was obtained on a patient receiving TMT to verify alignment before radiation treatment. In each panel, the cone beam CT image is in the upper left and bottom right portion of the image and the planning CT image is in the upper right and lower left portion. Note that image quality of cone beam CT is inferior to that of the diagnostic image. Overlay of the images allows comparison of the anatomy between scans to verify alignment of bony and soft-tissue structures. Transverse, sagittal, and coronal reconstructions are presented.

Table 2
Prospective trials of bladder preservation

Trial	Phase/Design	Stage	Number	Radiation (Gy)	Neoadjuvant Chemotherapy	Concurrent Chemotherapy	Adjuvant Chemotherapy	Complete Response	Bladder intact survival	5-y Overall Survival	Reference
BC2001	III	T2-T4a	360	55 of 64		5FU and Mitomycin				48%	James et al,[19] 2012
RTOG 02-33	Randomized phase II	T2-4a	93	40.3 + 24		Paclitaxel/ Cisplatin 5FU/Cisplatin	Cisplatin gemcitabine paclitaxel × 4	72% Pac 62% 5FU	67% paclitaxel 71% 5FU	71% paclitaxel 75% 5FU	Mitin et al,[24] 2013
RTOG 99-06	I/II	T2-T4a	80	40.3 + 24		Cisplatin + Paclitaxel	GC x 4	81	47%	56%	Kaufman et al,[23] 2009
RTOG 97-06	I/II	T2-T4a	46	40.8 + 24		Cisplatin	MCV x 3	74	47 (3 y)	61 (3 y)	Hagan et al,[6] 2003
RTOG 95-06	I/II	T2-T4a	34	24 + 40		Cisplatin + 5-FU		67	66 (3 y)	83 (3 y)	Kaufman et al,[22] 2000
RTOG 89-03	III	T2-T4a	123	39.6 + 25.2	MCV × 2 None	Cisplatin		61 51	36 40	49 48	Shipley et al,[12] 1998
RTOG 88-02	II	T2-T4a	91	39.6 + 25.2	MCV × 2	Cisplatin		75	44 (4 y)	62 (4 y)	Tester et al,[7] 1996
RTOG 85-12	II	T2-T4	42	40 + 24		Cisplatin		66		52	Tester et al (25)
Erlangan	N/A	T1-T4	415 (89 T1)	Median 54 (45-69.4)		Various: cisplatin, carboplatin, cisplatin + 5-FU		72	42	51%	Rodel et al,[4] 2002
MGH	N/A	T2-T4a	106	39.6 + 25.2	MCV × 2	Cisplatin		66	43	52	Kachnic et al,[11] 1997
Paris	N/A	T2-T4	54	24 +20		Cisplatin + 5-FU		74		59 (3 y)	Housset et al (53)
Italy	N/A	T2-T4	121	Median 65 (34-57)	MCV × 2	Cisplatin or carboplatin		86	51	68	Perdona et al,[9] 2008

Data from Refs.[4,6,7,9,11,12,22–25,53]

leads to a CR in approximately 70% of patients.[3] The 5-year OS and disease-specific survival with TMT in a series of prospective RTOG trials were 57% and 71%, respectively.[3] An intact bladder is preserved in approximately 80% of patients alive at 5 years after TMT.[3]

An important consideration is the ability of TMT to preserve a functional bladder. Although data are limited, single-institution studies suggest normal bladder function in 75% of conserved bladders as assessed by questionnaire and urodynamic studies.[18] A series of 112 patients treated with TMT-based bladder preservation reported that 79% of survivors with an intact bladder were delighted or pleased with urinary function.[44] The need for cystectomy to deal with complications of RT is uncommon and ranges from 0% to 2% in several series,[3,4,44,45] although bladder contracture not requiring cystectomy is reported in a subset of patients.

Other possible complications of TMT include gastrointestinal complaints and sexual dysfunction. The rate of these complications varies greatly by study, largely because of the method of collection of data. A review of late toxicity in 157 patients treated on RTOG trials who survived at least 2 years from the initiation of treatment found RTOG/EORTC (European Organisation for the Research and Treatment of Cancer) grade 3 late genitourinary toxicity in 5.7% and RTOG/EORTC grade 3 late gastrointestinal toxicity in 1.9%.[46] No grade 4 or 5 toxicities were reported in this series. Single-institution series using patient questionnaires have reported gastrointestinal complaints of any severity (10%–32% of patients) and sexual dysfunction (8%–38%) in a greater number of patients.[18,47,48]

Posttherapy surveillance remains a critical component of bladder preservation with TMT. Approximately 60% of recurrences after TMT are CIS and arise at the site of the original invasive tumor.[16] The risk of noninvasive failure is higher in patients with a component of CIS in the original tumor. Conservative management of these patients, with TURBT and intravesicle therapy, is recommended. Invasive recurrence is managed with salvage cystectomy.

Special Considerations

Response after induction

The presence of a CR to induction TMT is associated with an excellent long-term likelihood of bladder preservation. Obtaining less than a CR after induction therapy and undergoing immediate RC does not affect OS compared with those who require RC for late recurrences after achieving a CR. There are data to support that less than a CR to a complete course of TMT is associated with worse outcomes despite immediate RC, suggesting that reassessment after about 40 Gy is important to detect nonresponders.[4,29]

Both RTOG 99-06 and RTOG 02-33 allowed patients with a near-CR, including Tis and Ta, at the time of assessment following induction therapy to continue with definitive chemoradiation.[23,24] Among 119 patients in these trials, 85% achieved a T0 CR and 15% achieved a Ta or Tis (near-CR). This study was presented as an abstract[49] and showed that with a median follow-up of 5.9 years, 36% of patients with T0 tumor versus 28% of patients with Ta or Tis tumor experienced a bladder tumor recurrence (noninvasive and muscle invasive). Among 101 complete responders, 14 patients eventually required RC for salvage, in comparison with 1 patient among 18 near-complete responders ($P = .47$). There was no difference in disease-specific, bladder-intact, or overall survival. The investigators concluded that it is appropriate to recommend that patients with Ta or Tis tumor after induction TMT continue with bladder preservation. The numbers of patients included in this series are small, and confirmation will be useful.

Trimodality therapy for refractory/recurrent T1 disease

Bladder-preservation trials have focused on patients with MIBC; thus, data supporting TMT for T1 disease (lamina propria invasion) are limited. Treatment of T1 tumors typically involves conservative therapy with TURBT followed by intravesical bacillus Calmette-Guerin (BCG), with RC reserved for recurrent or refractory disease. Recent data indicate that concurrent chemoradiation may be an effective alternative to RC in patients with recurrent high-grade T1 tumors after failure of BCG treatment.[50,51]

One argument supporting the use of TMT for patients with refractory or recurrent high-grade T1 bladder tumors is the high rate of clinical-pathologic stage discrepancy. As many as 46% of patients with T1 disease who undergo RC are upstaged pathologically at surgery.[34] Given the high risk of occult MIBC in these patients, it has been suggested that more aggressive treatment with TMT may be warranted to avoid possible undertreatment.

The University of Erlangen reported their experience in 141 patients with high-risk T1 disease treated with bladder preservation as the initial treatment (80% received concurrent chemoradiation).[50] About 60% had T1 grade 3 (T1G3) disease; the others were high risk because of multifocal disease or CIS. Overall, there was an 88% CR rate and a progression rate of 19%. Of the patients with T1G3 tumors, the 10-year progression-free rate of the bladder tumor was 71% and 10-year disease-specific survival was 70%. This result compares favorably to most contemporary series of patients with T1G3 treated with TURBT and BCG.

A multicenter trial conducted in the United Kingdom evaluated whole-bladder radiation versus conservative therapy (observation or BCG depending on risk factors) after visibly complete TURBT in patients with previously untreated T1G3 bladder cancer to determine the efficacy of radiation in reducing the incidence of progression to MIBC.[52] There was no evidence of an advantage to the addition of radiation alone (no chemotherapy) in progression-free interval, progression-free survival, or OS. A complete TURBT was not required before radiation therapy, which may explain the higher-than-expected rates of recurrence. Although this trial suggested that RT alone may not be better than the current standard of care, the role of RT alone or concurrent with chemotherapy for recurrent disease after failure of BCG is undefined.

As previously noted, a wealth of data including 2 randomized trials demonstrate significantly better outcomes with the addition of radiosensitizing concurrent chemotherapy in the setting of bladder preservation in patients with MIBC. The current RTOG 0926 phase II trial is evaluating the role of bladder preservation with concurrent chemoradiation (cisplatin or 5-FU with MMC with 61.2 Gy) in operable patients with T1G3 disease in whom RC is the next conventional step in therapy.

Future Directions

Bladder preservation with TMT continues to evolve with refinements in radiation techniques and chemotherapy delivery. Improved ability to visualize and target the bladder tumor promises to minimize the margin of normal tissue treated, and, as a result, to minimize toxicity. Novel targeted agents are being explored to reduce the risk of distant failure and to enhance the local effects of RT. Enrollment of patients interested in TMT bladder preservation on clinical trials is important.

Patient selection for bladder preservation has to this point largely been accomplished by reviewing patient and tumor-related factors that predict for outcome after TMT. Several prognostic and predictive biomarkers that may allow improved patient selection and avoidance of TMT in patients at high risk of bladder tumor recurrence have been described.[31,53] Several markers have been explored in this context; however, most marker studies are most predictive of distant metastases and cause-specific survival, suggesting that they may have prognostic, not predictive, efficacy.[31,53] One notable exception is expression of Mre11, which is predictive for cause-specific survival after radical RT.[54] The identification of such markers may allow selection of therapy most appropriate based on rates of expected control with each treatment option.

REFERENCES

1. Siegel R, Ma J, Zou Z, et al. Cancer statistics, 2014. CA Cancer J Clin 2014;64:9–29.
2. Clark PE, Agarwal N, Biagioli MC, et al. Bladder cancer. J Natl Compr Canc Netw 2013;11:446–75.
3. Mak RH, Hunt D, Shipley WU, et al. Long-term outcomes in patients with muscle-invasive bladder cancer after selective bladder-preserving combined-modality therapy: a pooled analysis of radiation therapy oncology group protocols 8802, 8903, 9506, 9706, 9906, and 0233. J Clin Oncol 2014;32:3801–9.
4. Rodel C, Grabenbauer GG, Kuhn R, et al. Combined-modality treatment and selective organ preservation in invasive bladder cancer: long-term results. J Clin Oncol 2002;20:3061–71.
5. Efstathiou JA, Spiegel DY, Shipley WU, et al. Long-term outcomes of selective bladder preservation by combined-modality therapy for invasive bladder cancer: the MGH experience. Eur Urol 2012;61: 705–11.
6. Hagan MP, Winter KA, Kaufman DS, et al. RTOG 97-06: initial report of a phase I-II trial of selective bladder conservation using TURBT, twice-daily accelerated irradiation sensitized with cisplatin, and adjuvant MCV combination chemotherapy. Int J Radiat Oncol Biol Phys 2003;57:665–72.
7. Tester W, Caplan R, Heaney J, et al. Neoadjuvant combined modality program with selective organ preservation for invasive bladder cancer: results of Radiation Therapy Oncology Group phase II trial 8802. J Clin Oncol 1996;14:119–26.
8. Tester W, Porter A, Asbell S, et al. Combined modality program with possible organ preservation for invasive bladder carcinoma: results of RTOG protocol 85-12. Int J Radiat Oncol Biol Phys 1993; 25:783–90.
9. Perdona S, Autorino R, Damiano R, et al. Bladder-sparing, combined-modality approach for muscle-invasive bladder cancer: a multi-institutional, long-term experience. Cancer 2008; 112:75–83.
10. Shen SS, Lerner SP, Muezzinoglu B, et al. Prostatic involvement by transitional cell carcinoma in patients with bladder cancer and its prognostic significance. Hum Pathol 2006;37:726–34.

11. Kachnic LA, Kaufman DS, Heney NM, et al. Bladder preservation by combined modality therapy for invasive bladder cancer. J Clin Oncol 1997;15:1022–9.

12. Shipley WU, Winter KA, Kaufman DS, et al. Phase III trial of neoadjuvant chemotherapy in patients with invasive bladder cancer treated with selective bladder preservation by combined radiation therapy and chemotherapy: initial results of Radiation Therapy Oncology Group 89-03. J Clin Oncol 1998;16:3576–83.

13. Gospodarowicz MK, Hawkins NV, Rawlings GA, et al. Radical radiotherapy for muscle invasive transitional cell carcinoma of the bladder: failure analysis. J Urol 1989;142:1448–53 [discussion: 1453–4].

14. Wolf H, Olsen PR, Hojgaard K. Urothelial dysplasia concomitant with bladder tumours: a determinant for future new occurrences in patients treated by full-course radiotherapy. Lancet 1985;1:1005–8.

15. Fung CY, Shipley WU, Young RH, et al. Prognostic factors in invasive bladder carcinoma in a prospective trial of preoperative adjuvant chemotherapy and radiotherapy. J Clin Oncol 1991;9:1533–42.

16. Zietman AL, Grocela J, Zehr E, et al. Selective bladder conservation using transurethral resection, chemotherapy, and radiation: management and consequences of Ta, T1, and Tis recurrence within the retained bladder. Urology 2001;58:380–5.

17. Milosevic M, Gospodarowicz M, Zietman A, et al. Radiotherapy for bladder cancer. Urology 2007;69:80–92.

18. Zietman AL, Sacco D, Skowronski U, et al. Organ conservation in invasive bladder cancer by transurethral resection, chemotherapy and radiation: results of a urodynamic and quality of life study on long-term survivors. J Urol 2003;170:1772–6.

19. James ND, Hussain SA, Hall E, et al. Radiotherapy with or without chemotherapy in muscle-invasive bladder cancer. N Engl J Med 2012;366:1477–88.

20. Coppin CM, Gospodarowicz MK, James K, et al. Improved local control of invasive bladder cancer by concurrent cisplatin and preoperative or definitive radiation. The National Cancer Institute of Canada Clinical Trials Group. J Clin Oncol 1996;14:2901–7.

21. Krause FS, Walter B, Ott OJ, et al. 15-year survival rates after transurethral resection and radiochemotherapy or radiation in bladder cancer treatment. Anticancer Res 2011;31:985–90.

22. Kaufman DS, Winter KA, Shipley WU, et al. The initial results in muscle-invading bladder cancer of RTOG 95-06: phase I/II trial of transurethral surgery plus radiation therapy with concurrent cisplatin and 5-fluorouracil followed by selective bladder preservation or cystectomy depending on the initial response. Oncologist 2000;5:471–6.

23. Kaufman DS, Winter KA, Shipley WU, et al. Phase I-II RTOG study (99-06) of patients with muscle-invasive bladder cancer undergoing transurethral surgery, paclitaxel, cisplatin, and twice-daily radiotherapy followed by selective bladder preservation or radical cystectomy and adjuvant chemotherapy. Urology 2009;73:833–7.

24. Mitin T, Hunt D, Shipley WU, et al. Transurethral surgery and twice-daily radiation plus paclitaxel-cisplatin or fluorouracil-cisplatin with selective bladder preservation and adjuvant chemotherapy for patients with muscle invasive bladder cancer (RTOG 0233): a randomised multicentre phase 2 trial. Lancet Oncol 2013;14:863–72.

25. Tester W, Porter A, Asbell S, et al. Combined modality program with possible organ preservation for invasive bladder carcinoma: results of RTOG protocol 85-12. Int J Radiat Oncol Biol Phys 1993;25:783–90.

26. Kent E, Sandler H, Montie J, et al. Combined-modality therapy with gemcitabine and radiotherapy as a bladder preservation strategy: results of a phase I trial. J Clin Oncol 2004;22:2540–5.

27. Grossman HB, Natale RB, Tangen CM, et al. Neoadjuvant chemotherapy plus cystectomy compared with cystectomy alone for locally advanced bladder cancer. N Engl J Med 2003;349:859–66.

28. Sherif A, Holmberg L, Rintala E, et al. Neoadjuvant cisplatinum based combination chemotherapy in patients with invasive bladder cancer: a combined analysis of two Nordic studies. Eur Urol 2004;45:297–303.

29. Ploussard G, Daneshmand S, Efstathiou JA, et al. Critical analysis of bladder sparing with trimodal therapy in muscle-invasive bladder cancer: a systematic review. Eur Urol 2014;66:120–37.

30. Bolenz C, Shariat SF, Karakiewicz PI, et al. Human epidermal growth factor receptor 2 expression status provides independent prognostic information in patients with urothelial carcinoma of the urinary bladder. BJU Int 2010;106:1216–22.

31. Chakravarti A, Winter K, Wu CL, et al. Expression of the epidermal growth factor receptor and Her-2 are predictors of favorable outcome and reduced complete response rates, respectively, in patients with muscle-invading bladder cancers treated by concurrent radiation and cisplatin-based chemotherapy: a report from the Radiation Therapy Oncology Group. Int J Radiat Oncol Biol Phys 2005;62:309–17.

32. Michaelson MD, Hu C, Pham HT, et al. The initial report of RTOG 0524: phase I/II trial of a combination of paclitaxel and trastuzumab with daily irradiation or paclitaxel alone with daily irradiation following transurethral surgery for noncystectomy candidates with muscle-invasive bladder cancer. J Clin Oncol 2014;32(Suppl 4) [abstract: LBA287].

33. Goldsmith B, Baumann BC, He J, et al. Occult pelvic lymph node involvement in bladder cancer: implications for definitive radiation. Int J Radiat Oncol Biol Phys 2014;88:603–10.

34. Gray PJ, Lin CC, Jemal A, et al. Clinical-pathologic stage discrepancy in bladder cancer patients treated with radical cystectomy: results from the National Cancer Data Base. Int J Radiat Oncol Biol Phys 2014;88:1048–56.

35. Tunio MA, Hashmi A, Qayyum A, et al. Whole-pelvis or bladder-only chemoradiation for lymph node-negative invasive bladder cancer: single-institution experience. Int J Radiat Oncol Biol Phys 2012;82: e457–62.

36. Foroudi F, Pham D, Bressel M, et al. Intrafraction bladder motion in radiation therapy estimated from pretreatment and posttreatment volumetric imaging. Int J Radiat Oncol Biol Phys 2013;86:77–82.

37. Yee D, Parliament M, Rathee S, et al. Cone beam CT imaging analysis of interfractional variations in bladder volume and position during radiotherapy for bladder cancer. Int J Radiat Oncol Biol Phys 2010;76:1045–53.

38. Cowan RA, McBain CA, Ryder WD, et al. Radiotherapy for muscle-invasive carcinoma of the bladder: results of a randomized trial comparing conventional whole bladder with dose-escalated partial bladder radiotherapy. Int J Radiat Oncol Biol Phys 2004;59:197–207.

39. Mangar SA, Foo K, Norman A, et al. Evaluating the effect of reducing the high-dose volume on the toxicity of radiotherapy in the treatment of bladder cancer. Clin Oncol (R Coll Radiol) 2006;18:466–73.

40. Turgeon GA, Souhami L, Cury FL, et al. Hypofractionated intensity modulated radiation therapy in combined modality treatment for bladder preservation in elderly patients with invasive bladder cancer. Int J Radiat Oncol Biol Phys 2014;88:326–31.

41. Hsieh CH, Chung SD, Chan PH, et al. Intensity modulated radiotherapy for elderly bladder cancer patients. Radiat Oncol 2011;6:75.

42. Garcia MM, Gottschalk AR, Brajtbord J, et al. Endoscopic gold fiducial marker placement into the bladder wall to optimize radiotherapy targeting for bladder-preserving management of muscle-invasive bladder cancer: feasibility and initial outcomes. PLoS One 2014;9:e89754.

43. Baumgarten AS, Emtage JB, Wilder RB, et al. Intravesical lipiodol injection technique for image-guided radiation therapy for bladder cancer. Urology 2014; 83:946–50.

44. Weiss C, Engehausen DG, Krause FS, et al. Radiochemotherapy with cisplatin and 5-fluorouracil after transurethral surgery in patients with bladder cancer. Int J Radiat Oncol Biol Phys 2007;68: 1072–80.

45. Shipley WU, Kaufman DS, Zehr E, et al. Selective bladder preservation by combined modality protocol treatment: long-term outcomes of 190 patients with invasive bladder cancer. Urology 2002;60:62–7 [discussion: 67–8].

46. Efstathiou JA, Bae K, Shipley WU, et al. Late pelvic toxicity after bladder-sparing therapy in patients with invasive bladder cancer: RTOG 89-03, 95-06, 97-06, 99-06. J Clin Oncol 2009;27:4055–61.

47. Henningsohn L, Wijkstrom H, Dickman PW, et al. Distressful symptoms after radical radiotherapy for urinary bladder cancer. Radiother Oncol 2002;62: 215–25.

48. Caffo O, Fellin G, Graffer U, et al. Assessment of quality of life after cystectomy or conservative therapy for patients with infiltrating bladder carcinoma. A survey by a self-administered questionnaire. Cancer 1996;78:1089–97.

49. Mitin T, George A, Zietman AL, et al. Long-term outcomes among patients who achieve complete or near-complete responses after the induction phase of bladder-preserving combined modality therapy for muscle-invasive bladder cancer: a pooled analysis of RTOG 9906 and 0233. J Clin Oncol 2014; 32 [abstract: 284].

50. Weiss C, Wolze C, Engehausen DG, et al. Radiochemotherapy after transurethral resection for high-risk T1 bladder cancer: an alternative to intravesical therapy or early cystectomy? J Clin Oncol 2006;24: 2318–24.

51. Wo JY, Shipley WU, Dahl DM, et al. The results of concurrent chemo-radiotherapy for recurrence after treatment with bacillus Calmette-Guerin for non-muscle-invasive bladder cancer: is immediate cystectomy always necessary? BJU Int 2009;104: 179–83.

52. Harland SJ, Kynaston H, Grigor K, et al. A randomized trial of radical radiotherapy for the management of pT1G3 NXM0 transitional cell carcinoma of the bladder. J Urol 2007;178:807–13 [discussion: 813].

53. Housset M, Maulard C, Chretien Y, et al. Combined radiation and chemotherapy for invasive transitional-cell carcinoma of the bladder: a prospective study. J Clin Oncol 1993;11:2150–7.

54. Choudhury A, Nelson LD, Teo MT, et al. MRE11 expression is predictive of cause-specific survival following radical radiotherapy for muscle-invasive bladder cancer. Cancer Res 2010;70:7017–26.

Neoadjuvant Chemotherapy in the Management of Muscle-Invasive Bladder Cancer
Bridging the Gap Between Evidence and Practice

CrossMark

John P. Sfakianos, MD, Matthew D. Galsky, MD*

KEYWORDS

- Neoadjuvant chemotherapy • Muscle-invasive bladder cancer • Efficacy • Effectiveness

KEY POINTS

- Two randomized trials and a meta-analysis have demonstrated that neoadjuvant cisplatin-based combination chemotherapy results in an improvement in survival in patients with muscle-invasive bladder cancer.
- Physician-associated barriers, including concerns regarding delaying curative-intent surgery, have contributed to poor use rates of neoadjuvant cisplatin-based chemotherapy; thus, the development of novel perioperative regimens, which are highly active and can be administered safely and expediently, is of substantial interest.
- The widespread use of -omic platforms has improved the understanding of bladder cancer; this information is being used to form prediction models for response to cisplatin-based chemotherapy as well as the use of targeted agents.
- Novel immunologic therapies are showing promising activity, with a favorable safety profile, in patients with bladder cancer.

INTRODUCTION

In 2014, approximately 74,690 patients in the United States will be diagnosed with bladder cancer and approximately 15,580 patients will succumb to the disease.[1] Most patients will present with clinically localized disease. At initial presentation, muscle-invasive bladder cancer (MIBC) is present in approximately 30% of patients; approximately 8% to 10% of patients will have radiographic evidence of metastatic disease. MIBC is potentially curable, particularly with combined modality approaches. The fact that most patients do not have radiographic evidence of metastatic disease at the time of diagnosis affords a window of opportunity to eradicate local and micrometastatic disease. Unfortunately, even with the current approaches to curative-intent therapy for MIBC, approximately 50% of patients will still develop clinical evidence of distant metastasis and ultimately succumb to their disease in a median time of 14 months.[2–4]

Source of Funding: Not applicable.
Departments of Urology and Medicine, Icahn School of Medicine at Mount Sinai, 1 Gustave L Levy Place, New York, NY 10029, USA
* Corresponding author.
E-mail address: matthew.galsky@mssm.edu

urologic.theclinics.com

Novel therapeutic options for the management of bladder cancer have significantly lagged behind other malignancies. For example, since 1995, there has only been one new US Food and Drug Administration–approved therapy for the treatment of bladder cancer, an intravesical treatment of non–muscle-invasive disease. Although progress in the treatment of cancer should not be measured by drug approvals alone, this does provide at least one measurable metric of the state of the science. There are multiple potential reasons for this historical lack of progress, including a relatively poor understanding of disease biology, inadequate funding for research, and lack of investigator/industry interest in the disease.[5,6]

An important, but commonly overlooked, contributor to the lack of progress for the treatment of bladder cancer is the disconnect between the efficacy and the effectiveness of the gold standard treatments for the disease. The typical patient with bladder cancer often poorly resembles the patients enrolled on prospective clinical trials or included in single-center series from large academic medical centers. Acknowledging this gap, while simultaneously increasing our understanding of the pathogenesis of the disease, may ultimately lead to more effective treatments that can be safely applied to a larger proportion of patients with the disease.

NEOADJUVANT CHEMOTHERAPY AND RADICAL CYSTECTOMY: A GOLD STANDARD?

Although radical cystectomy with pelvic lymph node dissection is a mainstay of treatment of MIBC, several studies have demonstrated improved survival with cisplatin-based combination chemotherapy administered preoperatively. Two randomized trials and a meta-analysis have demonstrated an improvement in survival with neoadjuvant cisplatin-based chemotherapy before radical cystectomy in patients with MIBC.[7–9] The Southwestern Oncology Group (SWOG 8710) trial randomized patients with MIBC to 3 cycles of neoadjuvant methotrexate, vinblastine, doxorubicin plus cisplatin (MVAC) followed by radical cystectomy versus cystectomy alone.[8] The neoadjuvant chemotherapy arm demonstrated a median survival of 77 months versus 46 months with surgery alone (P = .06, 2-sided stratified log-rank test). Patients achieving a complete pathologic response fared best with an 85% survival rate at 5 years. Long-term data from a randomized trial of neoadjuvant cisplatin, methotrexate and vinblastine (CMV), followed by local therapy (either surgery or radiation) versus local therapy alone also demonstrated a survival benefit with the use of neoadjuvant chemotherapy (hazard ratio [HR]: 0.84; 95% confidence interval [CI], 0.72 to 0.99; P = .037) (**Table 1**). The benefit achieved with neoadjuvant cisplatin-based chemotherapy has been further supported by a meta-analysis of 3005 patients, demonstrating a 5% absolute improvement in survival at 5 years (HR: 0.86; 95% CI, 0.77–0.95; P = .003). Although several randomized trials have explored the use of adjuvant chemotherapy for bladder cancer, these studies have generally been flawed, underpowered, and/or prematurely terminated, yielding mixed results.

THE GAP BETWEEN EVIDENCE AND PRACTICE

Though radical cystectomy with neoadjuvant cisplatin-based chemotherapy is the gold standard for treatment of MIBC, both of these treatments have been shown to be vastly underused in population-based studies. In an analysis of Surveillance, Epidemiology, and End Results–Medicare data, Gore and colleagues[10] demonstrated that among 3262 patients aged 66 years and older with MIBC, only 21% underwent radical cystectomy. Similar results have been demonstrated in analyses using data from the National Cancer Database (NCDB), which represents data from greater than 70% of bladder cancer diagnoses in the United States. In an analysis of more than 28,000 patients from the NCDB, Gray and colleagues[11] found that only 52.5% of patients

Table 1			
Randomized clinical trials of neoadjuvant chemotherapy in MIBC			
Study	Number of Patients	Randomization	Outcomes
SWOG-8710	317	MVAC + surgery vs surgery alone	Overall survival improvement with MVAC (77 vs 46 mo; P = .06, 2-sided stratified log-rank test)
BA06 30894	976	CMV + surgery/radiation vs surgery/radiation alone	Risk reduction in overall survival by 16% with CMV (HR: 0.84; 95% CI, 0.72 to 0.99; P = .037)

with MIBC received aggressive therapy, defined as cystectomy, radiation, or chemoradiation. The use of aggressive therapy significantly decreased with advancing patient age (odds ratio: 0.34 for 81–90 years of age vs ≤50 years of age; $P<.001$).

As radical cystectomy is a major operation, with the potential for both treatment-related morbidity and mortality, the underutilization of this modality with advancing patient age is perhaps not surprising. Still, narrowing the gap between evidence and effectiveness requires establishing uniform definitions of cystectomy ineligibility, approaches to prehabilitate patients that are borderline cystectomy candidates, shared decision-making tools for choosing among the available curative local therapies (cystectomy vs radiation or chemoradiation), and standard-of-care regimens for patients who are neither candidates for cystectomy nor cisplatin-based concurrent chemoradiation.

Population-based analyses have also explored patterns of perioperative chemotherapy use for patients with MIBC and have begun to explore barriers to utilization. An analysis of an NCDB dataset of more than 7000 patients with MIBC identified that only 1.2% of patients received neoadjuvant chemotherapy and 10.4% received adjuvant chemotherapy.[12] Feifer and colleagues,[13] in collaboration with the Bladder Cancer Advocacy Network Muscle Invasive Bladder Cancer Quality of Care Consortium, performed a 2-phase evaluation of neoadjuvant chemotherapy use among a group of academic enters. In phase 1 of their study, they retrospectively evaluated 4972 patients and identified that neoadjuvant chemotherapy was administered in 12.4% of patients. A prospective phase 2 portion was subsequently initiated to define the precise reasons for the poor utilization of neoadjuvant chemotherapy, with the results pending. Booth and colleagues[14,15] explored the use of perioperative chemotherapy for MIBC using the Ontario Cancer Registry and reported that 4% of patients received neoadjuvant chemotherapy from 1994 to 2008. Notably, this group reported that only 18% (520 of 2944) of patients in the cohort were seen by a medical oncologist before cystectomy and that 25% of patients referred to a medical oncologist received neoadjuvant chemotherapy. There was marked geographic variation in medical oncology referral rates before cystectomy (5%–40%).

Decreased enthusiasm for the use of neoadjuvant chemotherapy, particularly in older patients, may be related, at least in part, to concerns regarding the toxicities associated with the regimens used in the neoadjuvant randomized trials, MVAC and CMV. In the metastatic setting, gemcitabine plus cisplatin (GC) has largely supplanted

MVAC as standard first-line therapy based on a phase III trial demonstrating similar efficacy albeit lesser toxicity.[16] These results have been extrapolated to the neoadjuvant setting and even included in the National Comprehensive Cancer Network's guidelines, in the absence of level I evidence, highlighting a pragmatic attempt by the oncology community to bridge the gap between efficacy and effectiveness. Retrospective studies have demonstrated similar complete pathologic rates comparing MVAC and GC, providing some support for this practice.[17] There are no randomized trials establishing the efficacy of perioperative carboplatin-based therapy for patients with MIBC and even scant prospective phase II data, leaving the large population of cisplatin-ineligible patients without a standard perioperative systemic therapy option.

As outlined earlier, barriers to the utilization of neoadjuvant chemotherapy for MIBC exist at the system-, physician-, and patient-levels. Comprehensively identifying and addressing each of these barriers, while simultaneously developing more effective and less toxic systemic therapies, are critical to optimizing the likelihood of cure of all patients with MIBC.

NEW APPROACHES TO PERIOPERATIVE CHEMOTHERAPY IN MUSCLE-INVASIVE BLADDER CANCER

Physician-related barriers to the integration of cisplatin-based neoadjuvant chemotherapy include concerns regarding toxicities potentially increasing cystectomy-related morbidity and mortality or even preventing surgery from proceeding at all. Several analyses exploring this issue have not supported these concerns. For example, in a study of 878 patients who underwent radical cystectomy from the American College of Surgeons National Surgical Quality Improvement Program database, on multivariate analysis, neoadjuvant chemotherapy was not associated with increased perioperative complications, need for reoperation, wound infection, or wound dehiscence.[18] Physicians have also raised concerns regarding delaying curative-intent surgery, while delivering potentially ineffective chemotherapy. Therefore, the development of novel perioperative regimens that are highly active and can be administered safely and expediently are of substantial interest.

Administering chemotherapy in a dose-dense fashion is based on the hypothesis that because cancer cells display Gompertzian growth kinetics, applying treatment at more frequent intervals may results in a higher log cell kill.[19] Sternberg and colleagues[20,21] developed a dose-dense MVAC regimen (ddMVAC) in patients with advanced bladder cancer and, though compared with standard-dose MVAC this regimen did not result in an improvement in median survival, ddMVAC was shown to potentially increase the likelihood of durable disease control in a subset of patients. Several recent studies have explored the use of ddMVAC in the neoadjuvant setting. In a phase II multicenter trial, Choueiri and colleagues[22] evaluated the activity of 4 cycles of neoadjuvant ddMVAC in 39 patients followed by radical cystectomy. In this single-arm study, ddMVAC was associated with a pathologic complete response rate of 49% (80% CI, 38%–61%) and with a 10% grade 3 or greater toxicity rate. In a similar study, 44 patients were treated with 3 cycles of neoadjuvant ddMVAC followed by radical cystectomy; 38% of patients achieved a pathologic complete response (95% CI, 25%–53%).[23] The regimen was reasonably well tolerated (12% of patient's experienced grade 3 or 4 toxicities).

Although these are relatively small single-arm trials, these studies do demonstrate that administration of ddMVAC with granulocyte colony stimulating factor support over a short time period (14-day cycles × 3–4) preoperatively is relatively safe and quite active (based on pathologic complete response rates). In fact, the National Comprehensive Cancer Network's practice guidelines now recommend dose-dense administration when MVAC is applied in the preoperative setting.

NEW APPROACHES TO INDIVIDUALIZE RISK PREDICTION

Another physician and patient barrier to implementation of neoadjuvant chemotherapy is the inability to identify individuals who most likely need treatment (ie, not be cured with surgery alone) and who are most likely to benefit from treatment (ie, harbor tumors sensitive to cisplatin-based chemotherapy). The use of high throughput -omic platforms has advanced the understanding of the heterogeneity of MIBC and offers the promise to refine our ability to individualize risk prediction. The use of gene expression profiling on MIBC samples has identified potential signatures of both patients at higher risk for metastatic disease as well as those less likely to respond to neoadjuvant cisplatin-based chemotherapy. Smith and colleagues[24] developed and validated a gene expression model to predict pathologic nodal status from primary tumor tissue in clinically node negative patients with the aim that this signature could ultimately be applied to transurethral resection specimens to identify patients most suitable for the integration of neoadjuvant chemotherapy.

This 20-gene signature was associated with an area under the curve of 0.67 (95% CI 0.60–0.75) for prediction of pathologic evidence of nodal disease at cystectomy and on multivariate logistic regression analysis was shown to be independent of clinical prognostic variables.

Recently, several independent groups have used gene expression profiling to identify distinct biologic subtypes of MIBC.[25,26] In an analysis from Choi and colleagues,[25] 3 subtypes of MIBC were identified: basal, luminal, and p53-like. Notably, the p53-like tumors were found to be resistant to cisplatin-based chemotherapy in 2 independent clinical datasets. This observation requires additional validation but is very compelling given both the biological and clinical significance of the findings.

Theodorescu and colleagues[28] have taken a novel approach to the development of gene signatures of chemotherapy sensitivity. The COXEN (Coexpression Extrapolation) bioinformatics algorithm uses gene expression and drug sensitivity data from a publically available cell line panel (National Cancer Institute 60 cell line panel), along with gene expression data from human tumors, to identify which genes are most commonly coexpressed.[27] A gene expression model is then developed to predict sensitivity to a single-agent or a multi-drug chemotherapeutic regimen. The COXEN model was retrospectively applied to a cohort of patients with bladder cancer treated with neoadjuvant MVAC and correlated with the likelihood of achieving tumor downstaging and 3-year overall survival.[27,28] Patients with a favorable COXEN score had a 3-year overall survival of 81% compared with those without a favorable score with a 3-year overall survival of 33% (P = .002).

Somatic mutations identified through next-generation sequencing efforts in bladder cancer specimens may also allow identification of patients most likely to benefit from cisplatin-based chemotherapy. For example, ERCC2, a nucleotide excision repair gene, was found to be mutated in 12% of MIBC specimens in The Cancer Genome Atlas (TCGA) analysis.[29] Following up on the clinical relevance of this observation, Van Allen and colleagues[30] performed whole-exome sequencing on 50 patients treated with neoadjuvant cisplatin-based chemotherapy, 25 responders and 25 nonresponders. Mutations in ERCC2 were significantly associated with a complete pathologic response. Plimack and colleagues[31] explored a panel of somatic mutations in DNA damage repair genes in the context of patients treated on their phase 2 trial of neoadjuvant ddMVAC. Intriguingly, they demonstrated that the pretreatment tumor specimens of all but one patient achieving a pathologic complete response to chemotherapy harbored mutations in *ATM*, *Rb1*, or *FANCC*, whereas none of the patients without a complete pathologic response harbored mutations in these genes.

Additional validation of all of these findings in a cohort of patients treated with neoadjuvant chemotherapy, with uniform specimen banking procedures, will be critical to advancing these biomarkers to clinical practice. Indeed, the recently opened SWOG randomized phase II trial (S1314) of neoadjuvant ddMVAC versus GC is designed with this very goal in mind. The trial will test the ability of the COXEN algorithm to predict pathologic complete response to these two chemotherapeutic regimens while also serving as a validation set for the association between chemotherapy sensitivity and the gene-expression-derived bladder cancer subsets and somatic mutations described earlier.

ALTERNATIVES TO CYTOTOXIC CHEMOTHERAPY IN THE PERIOPERATIVE SETTING?

The identification of novel targets, and novel approaches, to perioperative systemic therapy for MIBC may one day obviate cytotoxic chemotherapy and help bridge the gap between efficacy and effectiveness, particularly if associated with a more favorable therapeutic index. Modulating the host immune system to generate an antitumor immune response represents one potential attractive approach. A recently completed study explored the use of DN24-02, an autologous cellular immunotherapy product designed to stimulate an immune response against HER2/neu, as adjuvant therapy in patients with Her-2–expressing bladder cancer after cystectomy. Given the safety and tolerability of this approach, the results of this randomized phase II study are eagerly awaited.[32] Another promising approach to bladder cancer immunotherapy is to promote immune cell activation, specifically cytotoxic T cells, via blockade of key negative checkpoints, such as cytotoxic T lymphocyte–associated antigen (CTLA-4) and programmed cell death-1 (PD-1). In a window-of-opportunity presurgical study, Carthon and colleagues[33] treated 12 patients with ipilimumab, an anti-CTLA-4 antibody, before cystectomy. These investigators demonstrated that treatment was well tolerated and that cystectomy specimens from patients treated with a higher dose of ipilimumab harbored perivascular infiltrates of activated T cells. Ipilimumab is currently being further explored for the treatment of advanced bladder cancer. Blocking antibodies to PD-1 and PD ligand 1 (PD-L1) have emerged as particularly promising given their broad anticancer activity and generally favorable toxicity profile. Preliminary results of an expansion cohort in patients with bladder cancer enrolled on a phase I study of MPDL3280A (anti–PD-L1 antibody) have been reported.[34] This trial demonstrated relatively durable responses in a subset of patients with heavily pretreated metastatic bladder cancer with only 4% grade 3 to 4 adverse events. Furthermore, a correlation between PD-L1 expression on tumor-infiltrating cells by immunohistochemistry and response was reported: there was a 43% objective response rate for the PD-L1+ subset and an 11% objective response rate for PD-L1- subset. The exciting preliminary results of this trial, and other PD-1 and PD-L1 inhibitors, have led to the planning, or recent activation, of several trial integrating these antibodies in the perioperative setting.

Individualizing systemic therapies using small molecules directed at specific targets in patients' tumors is another potential approach to improving the therapeutic index of perioperative systemic therapy. The TCGA, a project funded by the National Cancer Institute and the National Human Genome Research Institute, performed comprehensive genomic profiling of a large cohort of MIBC specimens.[29] Intriguingly, the initial report from the TCGA bladder cancer analysis of 131 MIBC specimens identified that 69% of tumors harbored a potential therapeutic target. The safety and activity of targeting activating oncogenomic mutations in patients with metastatic bladder cancer is being established with 2 independent trials recently demonstrating proof of concept with small molecules directed against the fibroblast growth factor receptor in tumors harboring fibroblast growth factor receptor 3 alterations.[35] Applying these small molecules, and others, in appropriately selected patients in the perioperative setting is anticipated in the near future.

SUMMARY

Although cisplatin-based chemotherapy followed by radical cystectomy is the standard treatment of MIBC, population-based studies reveal that only a small fraction of patients with MIBC actually receive such treatment. A comprehensive understanding of the reasons for the gap between efficacy and effectiveness is necessary to narrow this disparity and increase the likelihood of cure of all patients with MIBC. These reasons include systems-, provider-, and patient-level barriers that are not amenable to a single solution. Tackling each barrier, while simultaneously advancing our understanding of the pathogenesis of the disease to improve the therapeutic index of cancer treatment, will ultimately be necessary to bridge the disconnect between what is *achievable* and what is actually *achieved*.

REFERENCES

1. Siegel R, Ma J, Zou Z, et al. Cancer statistics, 2014. CA Cancer J Clin 2014;64:9–29.
2. Bellmunt J, von der Maase H, Mead GM, et al. Randomized phase III study comparing paclitaxel/cisplatin/gemcitabine and gemcitabine/cisplatin in patients with locally advanced or metastatic urothelial cancer without prior systemic therapy: EORTC Intergroup Study 30987. J Clin Oncol 2012;30:1107–13.
3. Shariat SF, Karakiewicz PI, Palapattu GS, et al. Outcomes of radical cystectomy for transitional cell carcinoma of the bladder: a contemporary series from the Bladder Cancer Research Consortium. J Urol 2006;176:2414–22 [discussion: 22].
4. Stein JP, Lieskovsky G, Cote R, et al. Radical cystectomy in the treatment of invasive bladder cancer: long-term results in 1,054 patients. J Clin Oncol 2001;19:666–75.
5. Carter AJ, Nguyen CN. A comparison of cancer burden and research spending reveals discrepancies in the distribution of research funding. BMC Public Health 2012;12:526.
6. Galsky MD, Hendricks R, Svatek R, et al. Critical analysis of contemporary clinical research in muscle-invasive and metastatic urothelial cancer: a report from the Bladder Cancer Advocacy Network Clinical Trials Working Group. Cancer 2013;119:1994–8.
7. International Collaboration of Trialists, Medical Research Council Advanced Bladder Cancer Working Party, European Organisation for Research and Treatment of Cancer Genito-Urinary Tract Cancer Group, et al. International phase III trial assessing neoadjuvant cisplatin, methotrexate, and vinblastine chemotherapy for muscle-invasive bladder cancer: long-term results of the BA06 30894 trial. J Clin Oncol 2011;29:2171–7.
8. Grossman HB, Natale RB, Tangen CM, et al. Neoadjuvant chemotherapy plus cystectomy compared with cystectomy alone for locally advanced bladder cancer. N Engl J Med 2003;349:859–66.
9. Advanced Bladder Cancer Meta-analysis Collaboration. Neoadjuvant chemotherapy in invasive bladder cancer: update of a systematic review and meta-analysis of individual patient data advanced bladder cancer (ABC) meta-analysis collaboration. Eur Urol 2005;48:202–5 [discussion: 205–6].
10. Gore JL, Litwin MS, Lai J, et al. Use of radical cystectomy for patients with invasive bladder cancer. J Natl Cancer Inst 2010;102:802–11.
11. Gray PJ, Fedewa SA, Shipley WU, et al. Use of potentially curative therapies for muscle-invasive bladder cancer in the United States: results from the National Cancer Data Base. Eur Urol 2013;63:823–9.
12. David KA, Milowsky MI, Ritchey J, et al. Low incidence of perioperative chemotherapy for stage III bladder cancer 1998 to 2003: a report from the National Cancer Data Base. J Urol 2007;178:451–4.
13. Feifer A, Taylor J, Shouery M, et al. Multi-institutional quality-of-care initiative for nonmetastatic, muscle-invasive, transitional cell carcinoma of the bladder: phase I. J Clin Oncol 2011;29(Suppl 7) [abstract: 240].
14. Booth CM, Siemens DR, Li G, et al. Perioperative chemotherapy for muscle-invasive bladder cancer: a population-based outcomes study. Cancer 2014;120:1630–8.
15. Booth CM, Robert Siemens D, Peng Y, et al. Patterns of referral for perioperative chemotherapy among patients with muscle-invasive bladder cancer: a population-based study. Urol Oncol 2014;32(8):1200–8.
16. Dash A, Pettus JA, Herr HW, et al. A role for neoadjuvant gemcitabine plus cisplatin in muscle-invasive urothelial carcinoma of the bladder: a retrospective experience. Cancer 2008;113:2471–7.
17. Galsky MD, Harshman LC, Crabb SJ, et al. Comparative effectiveness of gemcitabine plus cisplatin (GC) versus methotrexate, vinblastine, doxorubicin, plus cisplatin (MVAC) as neoadjuvant therapy for muscle-invasive bladder cancer (MIBC). J Clin Oncol (Meeting Abstracts) 2014;32:4512.
18. Johnson DC, Nielsen ME, Matthews J, et al. Neoadjuvant chemotherapy for bladder cancer does not increase risk of perioperative morbidity. BJU Int 2014;114:221–8.
19. Simon R, Norton L. The Norton-Simon hypothesis: designing more effective and less toxic chemotherapeutic regimens. Nat Clin Pract Oncol 2006;3:406–7.
20. Sternberg CN, de Mulder PH, Schornagel JH, et al. Randomized phase III trial of high-dose-intensity methotrexate, vinblastine, doxorubicin, and cisplatin (MVAC) chemotherapy and recombinant human granulocyte colony-stimulating factor versus classic MVAC in advanced urothelial tract tumors: European Organization for Research and Treatment of Cancer Protocol no. 30924. J Clin Oncol 2001;19:2638–46.
21. Sternberg CN, de Mulder P, Schornagel JH, et al. Seven year update of an EORTC phase III trial of high-dose intensity M-VAC chemotherapy and G-CSF versus classic M-VAC in advanced urothelial tract tumours. Eur J Cancer 2006;42:50–4.
22. Choueiri TK, Jacobus S, Bellmunt J, et al. Neoadjuvant dose-dense methotrexate, vinblastine, doxorubicin, and cisplatin with pegfilgrastim support in muscle-invasive urothelial cancer: pathologic, radiologic, and biomarker correlates. J Clin Oncol 2014;32:1889–94.

23. Plimack ER, Hoffman-Censits JH, Viterbo R, et al. Accelerated methotrexate, vinblastine, doxorubicin, and cisplatin is safe, effective, and efficient neoadjuvant treatment for muscle-invasive bladder cancer: results of a multicenter phase II study with molecular correlates of response and toxicity. J Clin Oncol 2014;32:1895–901.

24. Smith SC, Baras AS, Dancik G, et al. A 20-gene model for molecular nodal staging of bladder cancer: development and prospective assessment. Lancet Oncol 2011;12:137–43.

25. Choi W, Porten S, Kim S, et al. Identification of distinct basal and luminal subtypes of muscle-invasive bladder cancer with different sensitivities to frontline chemotherapy. Cancer Cell 2014;25: 152–65.

26. Damrauer JS, Hoadley KA, Chism DD, et al. Intrinsic subtypes of high-grade bladder cancer reflect the hallmarks of breast cancer biology. Proc Natl Acad Sci U S A 2014;111:3110–5.

27. Lee JK, Havaleshko DM, Cho H, et al. A strategy for predicting the chemosensitivity of human cancers and its application to drug discovery. Proc Natl Acad Sci U S A 2007;104:13086–91.

28. Havaleshko DM, Cho H, Conaway M, et al. Prediction of drug combination chemosensitivity in human bladder cancer. Mol Cancer Ther 2007;6:578–86.

29. Cancer Genome Atlas Research Network. Comprehensive molecular characterization of urothelial bladder carcinoma. Nature 2014;507:315–22.

30. Van Allen EM, Mouw KW, Kim P, et al. Somatic ERCC2 mutations correlate with cisplatin sensitivity in muscle-invasive urothelial carcinoma. Cancer Discov 2014;4:1140–53.

31. Plimack ER, Dunbrack R, Brennan T, et al. Next-generation sequencing to identify molecular alterations in DNA repair and chromatin maintenance genes associated with pathologic complete response (pT0) to neoadjuvant accelerated methotrexate, vinblastine, doxorubicin, and cisplatin (AMVAC) in muscle-invasive bladder cancer (MIBC). J Clin Oncol (Meeting Abstracts) 2014;32:4538.

32. Bajorin DF, Gomella LG, Sharma P, et al. Preliminary product parameter and safety results from NeuACT, a phase 2 randomized, open-label trial of DN24-02 in patients with surgically resected HER2+ urothelial cancer at high risk for recurrence. J Clin Oncol (Meeting Abstracts) 2014;32:4541.

33. Carthon BC, Wolchok JD, Yuan J, et al. Preoperative CTLA-4 blockade: tolerability and immune monitoring in the setting of a presurgical clinical trial. Clin Cancer Res 2010;16:2861–71.

34. Harshman LC, Drake CG, Wargo JA, et al. Cancer immunotherapy highlights from the 2014 ASCO meeting. Cancer Immunol Res 2014;2:714–9.

35. Bahleda R, Dienstmann R, Adamo B, et al. Phase 1 study of JNJ-42756493, a pan-fibroblast growth factor receptor (FGFR) inhibitor, in patients with advanced solid tumors. J Clin Oncol (Meeting Abstracts) 2014;32:2501.

Radical Transurethral Resection Alone, Robotic or Partial Cystectomy, or Extended Lymphadenectomy

Can We Select Patients with Muscle Invasion for Less or More Surgery?

Eugene K. Cha, MD[a,1], Timothy F. Donahue, MD[b,c,1], Bernard H. Bochner, MD[a,*]

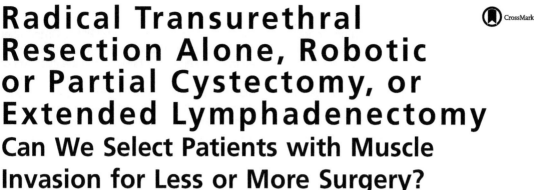

KEYWORDS

- Bladder-sparing • Bladder preservation • Radical transurethral resection • Partial cystectomy
- Extended lymphadenectomy

KEY POINTS

- Bladder-sparing approaches may be appropriate for select patients with muscle-invasive bladder cancer.
- In appropriately selected patients, outcomes for radical TUR and partial cystectomy may approach those achieved with radical cystectomy, but will require ongoing, long-term follow-up.
- Bladder-sparing approaches following neoadjuvant chemotherapy are currently limited by the inaccuracy of clinical staging and need further study.
- Some retrospective studies have reported associations between extended lymphadenectomy and improved clinical outcomes in patients treated with radical cystectomy and should be considered when surgically managing invasive bladder cancer.

INTRODUCTION

Radical cystectomy (RC) with pelvic lymph node dissection (PLND) remains the gold standard for local and regional therapy for muscle-invasive bladder cancer (MIBC),[1,2] with more contemporary standards including perioperative cisplatin-based chemotherapy.[3,4] For highly selected patients, surgical bladder preservation approaches including radical transurethral resection (TUR) and partial cystectomy (PC) with or without bilateral PLND may be reasonable alternatives to RC/PLND. A limited number of series have suggested that in appropriately selected patients, who represent a small fraction of all patients with MIBC, these approaches may offer reasonable oncologic outcomes while avoiding the morbidity associated with radical surgery[5] and body image issues associated with urinary diversion while simultaneously preserving

Disclosure statement: The authors have no relevant disclosures to report.
[a] Urology Service, Department of Surgery, Memorial Sloan Kettering Cancer Center, 353 East 68th Street, New York, NY 10065, USA; [b] Center for Prostate Disease Research, Uniformed Services University, 1530 East Jefferson Street, Rockville, MD 20852, USA; [c] John P. Murthy Cancer Center, Urology Service, Walter Reed National Military Medical Center, 8901 Rockville Pike, Bethesda, MD 20889, USA
[1] These authors contributed equally.
* Corresponding author. Urology Service, Department of Surgery, Kimmel Center for Prostate and Urologic Cancers, Memorial Sloan Kettering Cancer Center, 353 East 68th Street, New York, NY 10065.
E-mail address: bochnerb@mskcc.org

Urol Clin N Am 42 (2015) 189–199
http://dx.doi.org/10.1016/j.ucl.2015.02.003

urologic.theclinics.com

baseline urinary and sexual function. Furthermore, in the era of increasing perioperative systemic chemotherapy for MIBC, bladder-sparing approaches including radical TUR and PC have been investigated in patients demonstrating clinical response to neoadjuvant chemotherapy.

The multifocal nature of bladder cancer precludes many patients with MIBC from bladder-sparing surgical approaches. Two concepts have been proposed to account for bladder tumor multifocality.[6,7] The first, known as the "field defect" hypothesis, is that the entire urothelium is exposed to a variety of carcinogenic insults that result in independent tumors. The second is that multiple tumors arise from the spread of a single clone through intraepithelial migration or implantation.[8] Regardless of the cause, the multifocal nature of bladder tumors and recurrences needs to be taken into account when evaluating and considering bladder-sparing approaches to MIBC.

However, pathologic findings of no residual tumor at RC (pT0) suggest that there is a subset of patients who would be well-suited for bladder-sparing surgical approaches. The reported proportion of patients with a history of MIBC who achieve a pT0 response through TUR alone (without systemic neoadjuvant chemotherapy) ranges from 5% to 20% in the literature.[1,3,9] Although this identifies a subset of patients who might do well with surgical bladder-sparing therapies, approximately 7.5% of patients who achieve pT0 through TUR alone have LN-positive disease detected at time of RC/PLND, and a larger proportion of pT0 patients experience disease recurrence and ultimately death from bladder cancer.[3,9] In sum, although pT0 rates achieved through TUR alone suggest that there may be a subset of patients appropriate for surgical bladder-sparing approaches, the subset does not necessarily include all pT0 patients, nor can such patients be reliably identified. Clinical understaging remains a crucial obstacle to the successful implementation of bladder-sparing surgery for MIBC.

Regardless of the surgical technique used to manage invasive bladder cancer, regional pelvic LN spread is a known pathway of progression. Patients with non–muscle-invasive and pT2 disease at time of RC/PLND have a risk of LN involvement ranging from 5% to approximately 20%.[1,10] Although LN involvement represents a very strong negative prognostic finding, some patients with low-volume regional LN disease at time of RC/PLND experience long-term disease-free survival without further therapy. Strategies for the management of regional LN management for patients selected for bladder-sparing approaches have not been clearly established; most series of radical TUR or PC as definitive therapy for MIBC have eliminated or limited the extent of PLND. On the other end of the surgical spectrum, another arena for risk-adapted treatment of MIBC is the identification of patients for whom expanding the extent of surgery may be beneficial. Expanding the extent of lymphadenectomy in patients with MIBC being treated with RC/PLND improves the accuracy of staging and has a potential therapeutic benefit. Studies are ongoing to define the relationship between the extent of lymphadenectomy and disease progression, disease-specific survival, and overall survival.

BLADDER-SPARING APPROACHES FOR MUSCLE-INVASIVE BLADDER CANCER: RADICAL TRANSURETHRAL RESECTION

TUR, a diagnostic and therapeutic procedure in patients with non-MIBC, has been studied as a single-modality approach in patients with MIBC. Although the recurrence-free survival and long-term survival of unselected patients with muscle-invasive disease treated with TUR alone are inferior to those achieved by RC/PLND, in carefully selected patients, bladder-sparing approaches using radical TUR may be appropriate.

Historical series have reported relatively poor survival of patients with MIBC treated with TUR alone.[11–13] For example, in 1977, Barnes and colleagues[14] reported a 5-year survival rate of 31% for 75 patients exclusively undergoing TUR for the treatment of stage T2 bladder cancer. In contrast, Herr[15] reported that patients with muscle-invasive disease treated with radical TUR achieved a 5-year survival rate of 68%. However, only 45 of 217 patients were eligible for bladder-sparing treatment with radical TUR and 15 of these 45 patients (33%) were subsequently treated with RC or developed metastatic disease.

Henry and colleagues[16] reported a retrospective series comparing the outcomes of patients with stage B bladder cancer treated from 1974 to 1983 with TUR alone (N = 43), preoperative radiation and RC (N = 40), RC alone (N = 15), and definitive radiation therapy alone (N = 16). The 5-year survival rates for 43 patients with stages B1 and B2 disease treated with TUR were 63% and 38%, respectively; however, this was reported as comparable with survival rates in patients treated with radical surgery. Although the distribution of stage, grade, and number of tumors was not significantly different among the treatment groups, the sample size for each group was small and the groups were not randomized. For example, patients in the TUR groups were older and had more comorbidities than the other patients while having smaller tumors.

Selection of patients for bladder preservation with radical TUR is critical. A second or restaging

TUR (reTUR) provides an opportunity for more accurate staging in patients initially diagnosed with non-MIBC, allows for assessment of the completeness of the initial resection in patients with muscle-invasive disease, and provides important information regarding patient selection. In a study by Herr,[17] reTUR in 96 patients with non–muscle-invasive tumors revealed residual non–muscle-invasive disease in 55% and upstaging to T2 disease in 20%. Furthermore, in 54 patients with muscle-invasive disease at first TUR, 12 (22%) had no residual tumor and 30 (56%) had residual T2 disease.

Herr[18] further reported on the 10-year outcomes of 151 consecutive patients with MIBC who were offered bladder preservation with radical TUR after reTUR demonstrated no tumor (T0), residual carcinoma in situ (Tis), or non–muscle-invasive (T1) tumor and followed for at least 10 years. Of these 151 patients, 52 elected for immediate RC and 99 elected for bladder preservation. Of the 52 patients who elected immediate RC (all of whom had T0, Tis, or T1 disease on reTUR), 35% were upstaged to pT2, pT3, or pN+ on final pathology, highlighting the problem of clinical understaging. Of the 99 patients treated with TUR alone, 75 (76%) were alive at last follow-up and 24 (24%) died of disease, rates comparable with those treated with RC (71% alive and 29% dead of disease). Analysis revealed that 18% of patients who had T0 on reTUR died of bladder cancer compared with 42% of those who had T1 on reTUR ($P = .003$). The author concluded that the finding of residual T1 disease on reTUR be used to exclude patients from consideration of a radical TUR approach.

Solsona and colleagues[19,20] have reported results from a prospective study of 133 patients with MIBC treated with a macroscopically complete radical TUR who had negative biopsies of the tumor bed. They excluded patients with macroscopically residual tumor after TUR, hydronephrosis, clinical evidence of LN involvement, and distant metastatic disease. Additionally, tumors with a sessile appearance or those larger than 3 cm were excluded from the study. Long-term results from their study included cancer-specific survival rates of 81.9%, 79.5%, and 76.7% and progression-free survival of 75.5%, 64.9%, and 57.8% at 5, 10, and 15 years, respectively.[20] Approximately 30% of the patients in their study experienced disease progression, 22.5% as local bladder progression alone, 2.2% as local bladder progression associated with metastasis, and 5.5% as distant metastasis alone. Disease progression was associated with a high death rate of 67.5%, because only 12 patients were treated with salvage RC. Although 10 of the 12 patients treated with salvage RC (83.3%) were rendered free of disease, 89% of the remaining patients with disease progression who either refused or were not fit for salvage RC died of disease.

As demonstrated by the previously mentioned reports,[18,20] radical TUR may be an option for highly select patients (excluding those with residual T1 disease on reTUR, sessile lesions, or tumors >3 cm) with MIBC desiring bladder preservation (**Table 1**). Paramount to the success of radical TUR is the quality of initial TUR and reTUR. Furthermore, the patient and the physician must be dedicated to an intense and life-long regimen of endoscopic and radiographic surveillance. A major obstacle to the success of these approaches remains the inaccuracy of clinical staging, including the limitations of axial and molecular imaging.[21] Given the limited information reported on pelvic progression in these series, it is difficult to assess the need for PLND in these select cohorts. Molecular imaging techniques have not yet matured to allow for accurate detection of primary or recurrent disease. The use of PET with computed tomography (CT) has been limited by urinary excretion, which limits the ability to detect tumors within the bladder; however, newer tracer agents with minimal urinary excretion, such as ^{11}C-choline, are being tested.[22] Currently, PET-CT has been most effective in staging and the detection of metastatic disease. Kibel and colleagues[23] performed a prospective study using ^{18}F-FDG PET-CT in 43 patients undergoing RC and reported a positive predictive value of 78%, negative predictive value of 91%, sensitivity of 70%, and a specificity of 94%, leading the authors to conclude PET-CT may play an important role in planning treatment before cystectomy. MRI is increasingly used in the staging and longitudinal follow-up of patients with bladder cancer; however, the role of newer functional MRI techniques has yet to be definitively determined. As axial and molecular imaging techniques continue to evolve, additional refinements in the selection of patients suitable for surgical bladder preservation strategies will improve outcomes as those with locally advanced or occult regional disease can be identified and excluded. Long-term follow-up of additional prospective studies with clear patient selection criteria is needed for the critical evaluation of radical TUR as an option for select patients with MIBC.

BLADDER-SPARING APPROACHES FOR MUSCLE-INVASIVE BLADDER CANCER: PARTIAL CYSTECTOMY

PC represents an alternative surgical approach to bladder preservation with the advantages of

Table 1
Contemporary series of surgical bladder-sparing approaches for patients with muscle-invasive bladder cancer

Radical TUR	Eligibility Criteria	Cohort Size	Follow-Up	Outcomes	Notes
Herr,[18] 2001	Muscle-invasive bladder cancer Noninvasive disease on reTUR	Radical TUR: N = 99 Immediate RC: N = 52	Range: 10–20 y	Alive at last follow-up: 75 (76%) Died of disease: 24 (24%)	Patients with T0 on reTUR had better outcomes than those with T1 (CSS 82% vs 58%, respectively) 35% of patients electing immediate RC upstaged to pT2, pT3, pN+
Solsona et al,[19] 1998 Solsona et al,[20] 2010	Muscle-invasive bladder cancer Macroscopically complete radical TUR Negative biopsy of tumor bed Nonsessile appearance Tumor size ≤3 cm	N = 133	Mean: 112.1 mo Median: 99 mo Range: 11–305 mo	Recurrence: 40 (30%) Progression: 40 (30%) Died of disease: 27 (20%) Alive without tumor: 14 (11%) OS at 5, 10 y: 74%, 40% CSS at 5, 10 y: 82%, 80%	Progression associated with high death rate (67.5%) Highly select group (T0 by TUR alone)

Partial Cystectomy	Eligibility Criteria	Cohort Size	Follow-Up	Outcomes	Notes
Holzbeierlein et al,[30] 2004	Partial cystectomy for primary bladder tumor of nonurachal origin	N = 58	Mean: 33.4 mo Median: 31.3 mo Range: 1–82 mo	Died of disease: 12 (21%) OS at 5 y: 69%	Only 34 (59%) had cT2N0M0 disease CIS and multifocality associated with superficial recurrence LNI and positive surgical margin associated with advanced recurrence
Kassouf et al,[31] 2006	Muscle-invasive bladder cancer Solitary tumor No concomitant CIS No need for ureteral reimplantation	N = 37	Mean: 72.6 mo Median: 51 mo Range: 40–82 mo	Died of disease: 6 (16%) Died of other causes: 8 (22%) OS at 5 y: 67% CSS at 5 y: 87% RFS at 5 y: 39%	Adjuvant chemotherapy administered to 9 (24%) patients

Abbreviations: CIS, carcinoma in site; CSS, cancer-specific survival; LNI, lymph node involvement; OS, overall survival; RFS, recurrence-free survival.
Data from Refs.[18–20,30,31]

allowing for accurate staging through full-thickness examination of the primary tumor and the ability to perform a concurrent bilateral pelvic lymphadenectomy. As with radical TUR, patient and tumor selection are critical to the success of PC for the treatment of muscle-invasive disease.

Early experience with PC before the 1990s was marked by high recurrence rates, cancer recurrence within surgical wounds, and poor overall cancer control and survival. Historical series described local recurrence rates between 29% and 78%,[24,25] with 35% being noninvasive recurrences, 50% muscle-invasive recurrences, and 14% presenting with distant metastases.[26] Tumor recurrences within surgical incisions occurred in up to 40% of all patients and up to 54% in those with high-grade tumors.[24,27,28] Up to 20% of patients required salvage RC with 5-year overall survival rates of 50%.[29]

During the 1990s additional series from centers using strict selection criteria to identify appropriate candidates were reported.[30,31] These criteria include a solitary tumor in a location suitable for resection with a 2-cm margin of normal bladder, no associated carcinoma in situ, and no history of prior bladder tumors. Adequate bladder capacity and function should be maintained with the 2-cm margin of resection depending on initial bladder characteristics. Ureteral reimplantation, if necessary, is feasible. However, tumors located at the bladder neck or trigone may not be suitable for PC because achieving a suitable margin may be difficult. Using these more restrictive criteria, only 3% to 10% of patients presenting with muscle-invasive tumors remain candidates for PC.[30,31]

Retrospective analysis of 58 patients from Memorial Sloan Kettering Cancer Center (MSKCC) treated with PC (41 with muscle-invasive disease) identified that tumor multifocality ($P<.001$) and the presence of carcinoma in situ ($P = .027$) were associated with an increased risk of local recurrence following PC (see **Table 1**).[30] Pathologic confirmation of positive LNs and positive surgical margins were associated with advanced recurrences, defined as the development of recurrent muscle-invasive disease or distant metastases ($P = .012$ and $P = .022$, respectively). A study from MD Anderson reviewed 37 patients with muscle-invasive urothelial bladder cancer and demonstrated that history of prior bladder tumor ($P<.003$) was associated with disease recurrence.[31] Adjuvant chemotherapy may be considered for patients with pathologic evidence of extravesical disease or positive LNs after PC. In the series from MD Anderson, high-risk patients with locally advanced disease and positive LNs

treated with adjuvant chemotherapy (N = 9) had significantly longer progression-free survival, but overall and cancer-specific survival were not affected.[31] The ability to achieve an adequate negative surgical margin and adherence to these selection criteria cannot be overemphasized when evaluating a potential candidate for PC.

With refinements in patient selection, recurrence rates and overall survival in patients treated with PC have improved. Recurrence rates range from 28% to 48%; with non–muscle-invasive recurrence in 12% to 50%, muscle-invasive recurrence in 17% to 57%, and metastatic recurrence in 14% to 52%.[30–32] Positive surgical margins are described in 9% to 14% of patients undergoing PC; of the five patients with a positive surgical margin in the MSKCC series, three had muscle-invasive recurrence and one presented with distant metastases.[30] Salvage RC was required in 21% to 28% of patients,[30–32] with one series describing 75% of patients with muscle-invasive recurrences rendered disease-free after salvage RC.[31] The lack of wound recurrences and tumor implantation in these series is notable and likely reflective of appropriate patient selection and improvements in surgical technique.

These contemporary series report 5-year overall survival rates of 67% to 70%, recurrence-free survival rates of 39% to 62%, and cancer-specific survival rates of 84% to 87%.[30–32] Between 65% and 74% of patients maintained an intact bladder and 49% to 67% were free of disease with an intact bladder at last follow-up.[30,31] Although 86% of recurrences were described in the first 2 years after PC, late muscle-invasive recurrences have been reported indicating the need for lifelong surveillance in these patients.[31,32] Furthermore, these series have relatively short follow-up in comparison with mature RC series. As learned from the long-term follow-up from the Solsona series of radical TUR, longer follow-up is crucial to the evaluation of these results because patients remain at risk of recurrence and progression.

Contralateral nodal involvement in bladder cancer is not uncommon and is important when considering PLND for patients undergoing PC. Leissner and coworkers[33] reported on 119 patients whose bladder tumors could be strictly localized to one side of the bladder and found a significant rate of contralateral LN involvement with the risk of contralateral LN metastases only slightly lower than for the ipsilateral side. Furthermore, of 13 patients with unilateral tumors and a solitary LN metastasis, 3 of 13 (23%) of the solitary positive LNs were located on the contralateral side. The aforementioned series of PC did not explicitly describe the extent and laterality of the

PLNDs performed.[30,31] Nevertheless, 9% and 14% of the patients in the MSKCC and MD Anderson series had positive LNs, respectively; this proportion might be higher if all patients were treated with bilateral PLND. Currently, the accuracy of axial and molecular imaging and the ability to predict which patients have occult LN metastases are limited.[23,34] Patients undergoing a PLND at the time of PC should have a bilateral node dissection performed for accuracy of staging and added potential therapeutic advantage in the setting of limited pelvic nodal involvement.

Minimally invasive approaches are being investigated and adopted for a variety of urologic oncologic surgeries, including RC for bladder cancer.[35–37] Similarly, robot-assisted PC might represent an alternative to open PC.[38] Surgeons must maintain strict adherence to oncologic principles as the techniques of minimally invasive PC are refined and outcomes should be critically analyzed before widespread adoption of the procedure.

BLADDER-SPARING APPROACHES FOR MUSCLE-INVASIVE BLADDER CANCER FOLLOWING NEOADJUVANT CHEMOTHERAPY

With the demonstration of benefit and subsequent increased use of neoadjuvant chemotherapy for MIBC,[3] various investigators have explored the option for bladder-sparing techniques in patients demonstrating clinical responses to chemotherapy.

Herr and colleagues[39] reported results of 111 consecutive patients with MIBC treated with methotrexate, vinblastine, adriamycin, and cisplatin (MVAC) chemotherapy. Of the 111 patients, 50 (54%) had a complete clinical response (tumor site biopsy negative and urine cytology negative) as evaluated by postchemotherapy TUR. Although all of these patients were advised to undergo RC or PC, 28 refused surgery and were managed with TUR alone, 15 were treated with PC, and 17 elected treatment with RC. Although the number of patients in each treatment arm was small and treatment assignment was not randomized, the authors reported no difference in metastasis-free survival at 10 years between the treatment groups (74% with TUR or PC, 65% with RC), although patients who elected RC had more advanced clinical stage prechemotherapy. Of the 43 patients who were treated either with TUR alone or PC, 25 (58%) retained their bladder beyond 10 years.

In a prospective trial conducted by Sternberg and coworkers,[40] 104 patients with MIBC underwent TUR of bladder tumor after three cycles of MVAC and 49% of the cohort achieved cT0 on restaging (TUR pathology and CT scan). Thirty-seven patients who achieved cT0 after chemotherapy were treated with TUR alone; 11 were treated for non–muscle-invasive recurrences and four underwent salvage RC. Nineteen patients (51%) who had a cT0 response remained alive at a median follow-up of 56 months. Thirteen patients with solitary tumors who responded to MVAC chemotherapy were treated with PC. Two patients (15%) developed non–muscle-invasive recurrences, and three patients (23%) developed locally invasive disease. The 5-year overall survival rate for patients treated with PC after MVAC was 69%.

These promising results led to a phase II trial (Southwest Oncology Group [SWOG] 0219) incorporating an option for cystoscopic surveillance following cT0 response to chemotherapy. In this trial, 77 patients were treated with paclitaxel, carboplatin, and gemcitabine; patients who achieved cT0 status following paclitaxel, carboplatin, and gemcitabine chemotherapy could elect immediate RC or cystoscopic surveillance.[41] Thirty-four of 74 evaluable patients (46%) achieved cT0 status. Of the 10 patients with cT0 who elected for immediate RC, six had persistent muscle-invasive disease. These poor results highlight the potential inaccuracy of clinical staging that hinders any approach to bladder-sparing therapy for MIBC.

Although bladder-sparing surgical therapy may remain an option for patients who exhibit a clinical complete response to neoadjuvant chemotherapy, the success of such an approach relies heavily on the accuracy of clinical staging. Clinical staging, consisting of bimanual examination under anesthesia, TUR of prior tumor sites, and axial imaging, has significant room for improvement. The safety and efficacy of either cystoscopic surveillance or PC for patients who achieve cT0 following neoadjuvant chemotherapy for MIBC should be further studied in additional prospective trials, particularly as the accuracy of molecular imaging improves.

EXTENDED LYMPHADENECTOMY FOR MUSCLE-INVASIVE BLADDER CANCER

Pathologic tumor (pT) stage and LN status have been shown to be the strongest prognostic factors in patients undergoing RC/PLND for bladder cancer.[1,2,42,43] Although the importance of the staging information provided by PLND is well accepted, the anatomic boundaries of the dissections required for adequate and optimal staging remain to be clarified. A lack of prospectively validated studies has led to ongoing controversy regarding the necessary extent of dissection and magnitude of therapeutic benefit conferred.[44]

Distribution of Lymph Node Metastases

The primary lymphatic drainage for the urinary bladder includes the internal iliac, external iliac, obturator, and presacral LNs. Secondary drainage progresses to the common iliac LNs and then into the paraaortic, interaortocaval, and paracaval nodes.[33,45,46] Several studies have examined the location of LN metastases based on different anatomic templates of dissection.

Wishnow and colleagues[47] studied the rate of involvement of the pelvic LNs within the common iliac, obturator, internal iliac, and external iliac LNs in patients with bladder cancer undergoing RC. In a series of 130 patients with clinically negative LNs at the time of RC, 88% of whom had common iliac LNs resected, 14% were identified to have nodal metastasis. Seventeen of the 18 LN-positive patients had only one or two positive LNs. None of the 17 patients with one or two microscopically involved LNs had involvement of the common iliac or lateral external iliac LNs. Based on these findings, the authors advocated limiting the proximal limit of the PLND to the bifurcation of the common iliac vessels for patients with no gross evidence of nodal involvement at the time of surgery.[47]

A multicenter, prospective trial in which all patients underwent an extended lymphadenectomy (proximal limit of dissection at or above the bifurcation of the aorta) provided additional information on the distribution of positive pelvic LNs.[33] Of the 290 patients in this study, 81 (28%) had tumor involvement in 599 pelvic LNs; 35% of all positive LNs were proximal to the bifurcation of the common iliac vessels. Twenty patients (6.9%) had common iliac LN involvement without evidence of disease in the more distal nodal regions (obturator, internal iliac, or external iliac). Furthermore, in the 29 patients with only a single nodal metastasis, 10% had the solitary positive LNs proximal to the bifurcation of the common iliac vessels, providing support for extending the dissection to at least include the common iliac chain.[33]

More recently at our institution, a series of 591 patients undergoing RC with extended mapping PLND identified 114 patients (19%) with LN involvement.[10] In the node-positive group, 42 patients (37%) had involvement of the common iliac LNs (pN3), so these patients would have been understaged had a standard PLND been performed. Even more dramatically, seven of these patients (17% of pN3 patients, 6% of node-positive group) had no positive LNs within the true pelvis, so they would have been classified as node-negative had they undergone a standard PLND. These data provide strong support for the need to extend the PLND to include the common iliac LNs to maximize the accuracy of nodal staging.[10]

Outcomes Based on Extent of Lymphadenectomy: Number of Lymph Nodes Removed

The number of LNs removed has been widely used as a surrogate for extent of lymphadenectomy and has been demonstrated to be an important prognostic factor in patients with bladder cancer undergoing RC/PLND.[10,33,48,49] However, the number of LNs reported depends not only on the quality, extent, and thoroughness of PLND, but also the packaging of specimens and pathologic processing.[50] Although the benefit of PLND in terms of oncologic outcomes was initially reported in LN-positive patients,[51] its value in LN-negative patients has also been suggested.[52]

Leissner and colleagues[53] studied 447 patients who underwent RC/PLND and reported an association between the number of LNs removed and clinical outcomes. A threshold value of 16 LNs removed was used because the correlation between the total number of LNs removed and the percentage of patients with positive LNs was strongest at this cutoff. The authors found significant differences in recurrence-free survival and cancer-specific survival between patients with 16 or more LNs removed and patients with less than 16 LNs removed.

Herr and coworkers[48] analyzed data on 322 patients with MIBC who underwent RC/PLND. The authors evaluated the associations between the number of LNs removed with local recurrence-free and overall survival. In both LN-negative and LN-positive cases, improved overall survival was associated with a greater number of LNs removed. Herr and colleagues[48] concluded that at least nine LNs should be removed to accurately define LN status.

May and colleagues[52] reported on 1291 LN-negative patients who underwent RC and PLND and found that a higher number of LNs removed was associated with improved cancer-specific survival. Similarly to Leissner and colleagues,[53] the authors defined an LN threshold of 16 and showed that patients with less than 16 and 16 or more LNs removed had 5-year cancer-specific survival estimates of 72% and 83%, respectively ($P = .01$).

The concern that patient selection may bias who receives a more extended PLND at RC led Koppie and colleagues[54] to control for a variety of factors in their analyses to minimize the effects of surgical selection. The authors found that older patients with a greater degree of comorbidities were less likely to undergo more extensive PLNDs. However, when correcting for age and comorbidity, reported LN number was still associated with cancer-specific outcomes. The authors demonstrated that the probability of overall survival continued to increase with a greater number of LNs removed.

Outcomes Based on Extent of Lymphadenectomy: Anatomic Limits of Dissection

Given the limitations and biases of studies examining the number of LNs removed, investigators have analyzed data regarding the impact of anatomically defined extended PLND on outcome in patients with bladder cancer. Poulsen and colleagues[55] compared two consecutive series of patients who underwent extended PLND up the aortic bifurcation with those who underwent standard PLND. The authors found that extended PLND was associated with improved 5-year probabilities for pelvic and distant recurrence-free survival in patients with less than or equal to pT3a disease.

A prospective, single-center nonrandomized study was performed by Abol-Enein and colleagues[56] to evaluate the effect of a defined extended lymphadenectomy on recurrence-free survival. Specimens from individual anatomic regions were packaged separately. An intraoperative decision to perform an extended PLND was based on the status of the liver, body mass index, and performance status. The authors found that an anatomically defined extended lymphadenectomy up to the level of the inferior mesenteric artery (IMA), compared with a standard PLND (endopelvic region composed of obturator, internal iliac, and external iliac LNs), was associated with an improved recurrence-free survival for LN-positive patients independent of other clinicopathologic factors.

Although no prospective randomized data are currently available comparing a standard PLND (bilateral external and internal iliac and obturator nodes) with a more extended PLND, studies have compared outcomes from institutions performing varying extents of PLND. Dhar and colleagues[57] reported a comparative study evaluating disease-specific outcomes in 336 patients from one institution who underwent RC with a more limited PLND (boundaries included the pelvic sidewall between the genitofemoral and obturator nerves, and bifurcation of the iliac vessels to the circumflex iliac vein) with 322 patients from another institution who underwent a more extensive PLND (cephalad extent extended to the crossing of the ureters with the common iliac

vessels and removal of all tissue along the lateral and medial portion of the internal iliac vessels) at RC. Patients who underwent a more extensive PLND were more likely to be LN-positive (improved staging) and demonstrated improved recurrence-free survival. Five-year disease-free survival for node-positive patients undergoing an extended PLND was 35% versus only 7% in patients that received a limited PLND. Furthermore, patients treated with a more extensive PLND were less likely to experience isolated local recurrence (4% extended vs 38% limited); this difference persisted when analyzing by pathologic subgroups (1% extended vs 19% limited in pT2N0 cases, and 7% extended vs 60% limited in pT3N0 cases).

A study by Zehnder and colleagues[58] compared outcomes at two separate institutions based on different templates of PLND; 405 patients underwent extended PLND (mid-upper third of common iliac) and 554 patients underwent superextended lymphadenectomy (up to the IMA). Patients who underwent superextended lymphadenectomy had a higher number of LNs removed, a higher number of positive LNs, and a higher rate of LN metastasis (35% vs 28%; $P = .02$) compared with those who underwent extended PLND. Despite these differences, the two groups had equal recurrence rates and similar 5-year recurrence-free survival when stratified by pathologic tumor stage or LN status.

Ongoing Randomized Studies Evaluating Extent of Lymphadenectomy

The aforementioned studies have provided some insights into how the extent of PLND affects the accuracy of staging and may have an effect on clinical outcomes. However, there exists no high-level evidence to define the relationship between the extent of lymphadenectomy and disease progression, disease-specific survival, and overall survival. To that end, there are two ongoing clinical trials designed to address this question (**Table 2**).

The Association of Urogenital Oncology and the German Cancer Association have completed accrual to a phase 3 trial comparing extended PLND (up to the IMA) with conventional PLND (obturator, internal iliac, and external iliac LNs). The primary endpoint is progression-free survival; the study has 90% power to detect a 15% difference at 5 years. The results are yet to be reported.

The trial being performed by the SWOG 1011 is similarly designed but uses different assumptions and power calculations. The SWOG study has 85% power to detect a 28% reduction in the hazard rate of progression or death with extended

Table 2
Ongoing randomized clinical trials exploring benefit of extended lymphadenectomy at time of RC

	Accrual Goal	Extent of LN Dissection	Primary Endpoint/Power	Secondary Endpoints
Association of Urogenital Oncology and German Cancer Association	N = 450	Standard: external iliac, obturator, internal iliac LNs Extended: up to IMA	Progression-free survival at 5 y 90% power to detect a 15% difference	Local recurrence Distant metastases Disease-specific survival Complications
SWOG 1011	N = 620	Standard: external iliac, obturator, internal iliac LNs Extended: includes common iliac LNs and presacral LNs; can be extended up to IMA per surgeon preference	Disease-free survival 85% power to detect a 28% reduction in HR of progression or death	Overall survival Operative time Morbidity and mortality Length of hospital stay LN counts Local and retroperitoneal soft tissue recurrence

Abbreviations: HR, hazard ratio; IMA, inferior mesenteric artery.

PLND compared with conventional PLND. The trial is currently accruing patients, with a target of 620 patients.

These two important clinical trials should help to characterize the magnitude of clinical benefit that may be conferred by an extended PLND at RC and will provide additional data to help define appropriate standards of care. Given the previously reported rates of N3 involvement in the overall group of patients with MIBC, careful evaluation of the frequency of common iliac LN involvement in these studies will determine if they were adequately statistically powered to reach their primary endpoints.

SUMMARY

Anatomic and clinical studies of patients with bladder cancer have provided insights into the natural pathways of disease progression. Decades of experience with surgery for the management of MIBC clearly illustrates the role that surgical quality plays in patient outcomes. Improvements in the accuracy of clinical staging and further refinements in patient selection may allow for improved outcomes of bladder-preservation strategies incorporating radical TUR and PC with PLND. Well-designed and properly powered prospective clinical trials will provide the information necessary to establish whether disease-specific survival can be maintained with bladder preservation and improved with use of more extensive PLND at time of RC.

REFERENCES

1. Stein JP, Lieskovsky G, Cote R, et al. Radical cystectomy in the treatment of invasive bladder cancer: long-term results in 1,054 patients. J Clin Oncol 2001;19(3):666–75.
2. International Bladder Cancer Nomogram Consortium, Bochner BH, Kattan MW, et al. Postoperative nomogram predicting risk of recurrence after radical cystectomy for bladder cancer. J Clin Oncol 2006;24(24):3967–72.
3. Grossman HB, Natale RB, Tangen CM, et al. Neoadjuvant chemotherapy plus cystectomy compared with cystectomy alone for locally advanced bladder cancer. N Engl J Med 2003;349(9):859–66.
4. International Collaboration of Trialists, Medical Research Council Advanced Bladder Cancer Working Party (now the National Cancer Research Institute Bladder Cancer Clinical Studies Group), European Organisation for Research and Treatment of Cancer Genito-Urinary Tract Cancer Group, et al. International phase III trial assessing neoadjuvant cisplatin, methotrexate, and vinblastine chemotherapy for muscle-invasive bladder cancer: long-term results of the BA06 30894 trial. J Clin Oncol 2011;29(16):2171–7.
5. Shabsigh A, Korets R, Vora KC, et al. Defining early morbidity of radical cystectomy for patients with bladder cancer using a standardized reporting methodology. Eur Urol 2009;55(1):164–74.
6. Harris AL, Neal DE. Bladder cancer: field versus clonal origin. N Engl J Med 1992;326(11):759–61.
7. Habuchi T. Origin of multifocal carcinomas of the bladder and upper urinary tract: molecular analysis and clinical implications. Int J Urol 2005; 12(8):709–16.
8. Hafner C, Knuechel R, Zanardo L, et al. Evidence for oligoclonality and tumor spread by intraluminal seeding in multifocal urothelial carcinomas of the upper and lower urinary tract. Oncogene 2001; 20(35):4910–5.

9. Tilki D, Svatek RS, Novara G, et al. Stage pT0 at radical cystectomy confers improved survival: an international study of 4,430 patients. J Urol 2010; 184(3):888–94.

10. Tarin TV, Power NE, Ehdaie B, et al. Lymph node-positive bladder cancer treated with radical cystectomy and lymphadenectomy: effect of the level of node positivity. Eur Urol 2012;61(5):1025–30.

11. Flocks RH. Treatment of patients with carcinoma of the bladder. J Am Med Assoc 1951;145(5):295–301.

12. Milner WA. The role of conservative surgery in the treatment of bladder tumours. Br J Urol 1954;26(4):375–86.

13. O'Flynn JD, Smith JM, Hanson JS. Transurethral resection for the assessment and treatment of vesical neoplasms: a review of 840 consecutive cases. Eur Urol 1975;1(1):38–40.

14. Barnes RW, Dick AL, Hadley HL, et al. Survival following transurethral resection of bladder carcinoma. Cancer Res 1977;37(8 Pt 2):2895–7.

15. Herr HW. Conservative management of muscle-infiltrating bladder cancer: prospective experience. J Urol 1987;138(5):1162–3.

16. Henry K, Miller J, Mori M, et al. Comparison of transurethral resection to radical therapies for stage B bladder tumors. J Urol 1988;140(5):964–7.

17. Herr HW. The value of a second transurethral resection in evaluating patients with bladder tumors. J Urol 1999;162(1):74–6.

18. Herr HW. Transurethral resection of muscle-invasive bladder cancer: 10-year outcome. J Clin Oncol 2001;19(1):89–93.

19. Solsona E, Iborra I, Ricós JV, et al. Feasibility of transurethral resection for muscle infiltrating carcinoma of the bladder: long-term followup of a prospective study. J Urol 1998;159(1):95–8 [discussion: 98–9].

20. Solsona E, Iborra I, Collado A, et al. Feasibility of radical transurethral resection as monotherapy for selected patients with muscle invasive bladder cancer. J Urol 2010;184(2):475–80.

21. Vargas HA, Akin O, Schöder H, et al. Prospective evaluation of MRI, (1)(1)C-acetate PET/CT and contrast-enhanced CT for staging of bladder cancer. Eur J Radiol 2012;81(12):4131–7.

22. Maurer T, Souvatzoglou M, Kübler H, et al. Diagnostic efficacy of [11C]choline positron emission tomography/computed tomography compared with conventional computed tomography in lymph node staging of patients with bladder cancer prior to radical cystectomy. Eur Urol 2012;61(5):1031–8.

23. Kibel AS, Dehdashti F, Katz MD, et al. Prospective study of [18F]fluorodeoxyglucose positron emission tomography/computed tomography for staging of muscle-invasive bladder carcinoma. J Clin Oncol 2009;27(26):4314–20.

24. Faysal MH, Freiha FS. Evaluation of partial cystectomy for carcinoma of bladder. Urology 1979;14(4):352–6.

25. Merrell RW, Brown HE, Rose JF. Bladder carcinoma treated by partial cystectomy: a review of 54 cases. J Urol 1979;122(4):471–2.

26. Dandekar NP, Tongaonkar HB, Dalal AV, et al. Partial cystectomy for invasive bladder cancer. J Surg Oncol 1995;60(1):24–9.

27. Long RT, Grummon RA, Spratt JS Jr, et al. Carcinoma of the urinary bladder. Comparison with radical, simple, and partial cystectomy and intravesical formalin. Cancer 1972;29(1):98–105.

28. Peress JA, Waterhouse K, Cole AT. Complications of partial cystectomy in patients with high grade bladder carcinoma. J Urol 1977;118(5):761.

29. Kaneti J. Partial cystectomy in the management of bladder carcinoma. Eur Urol 1986;12(4):249–52.

30. Holzbeierlein JM, Lopez-Corona E, Bochner BH, et al. Partial cystectomy: a contemporary review of the Memorial Sloan-Kettering Cancer Center experience and recommendations for patient selection. J Urol 2004;172(3):878–81.

31. Kassouf W, Swanson D, Kamat AM, et al. Partial cystectomy for muscle invasive urothelial carcinoma of the bladder: a contemporary review of the M. D. Anderson Cancer Center experience. J Urol 2006; 175(6):2058–62.

32. Smaldone MC, Jacobs BL, Smaldone AM, et al. Long-term results of selective partial cystectomy for invasive urothelial bladder carcinoma. Urology 2008;72(3):613–6.

33. Leissner J, Ghoneim MA, Abol-Enein H, et al. Extended radical lymphadenectomy in patients with urothelial bladder cancer: results of a prospective multicenter study. J Urol 2004;171(1):139–44.

34. Karakiewicz PI, Shariat SF, Palapattu GS, et al. Precystectomy nomogram for prediction of advanced bladder cancer stage. Eur Urol 2006; 50(6):1254–60 [discussion: 1261–2].

35. Bochner BH, Sjoberg DD, Laudone VP, et al. A randomized trial of robot-assisted laparoscopic radical cystectomy. N Engl J Med 2014;371(4): 389–90.

36. Cha EK, Wiklund NP, Scherr DS. Recent advances in robot-assisted radical cystectomy. Curr Opin Urol 2011;21(1):65–70.

37. Bochner BH, Dalbagni G, Sjoberg DD, et al. Comparing open radical cystectomy and robot-assisted laparoscopic radical cystectomy: a randomized clinical trial. Eur Urol 2014. [Epub ahead of print].

38. Allaparthi S, Ramanathan R, Balaji KC. Robotic partial cystectomy for bladder cancer: a single-institutional pilot study. J Endourol 2010;24(2): 223–7.

39. Herr HW, Bajorin DF, Scher HI. Neoadjuvant chemotherapy and bladder-sparing surgery for invasive bladder cancer: ten-year outcome. J Clin Oncol 1998;16(4):1298–301.

40. Sternberg CN, Pansadoro V, Calabrò F, et al. Can patient selection for bladder preservation be based on response to chemotherapy? Cancer 2003;97(7): 1644–52.

41. deVere White RW, Lara PN Jr, Goldman B, et al. A sequential treatment approach to myoinvasive urothelial cancer: a phase II Southwest Oncology Group trial (S0219). J Urol 2009;181(6):2476–80 [discussion: 2480–1].

42. Hautmann RE, Gschwend JE, de Petriconi RC, et al. Cystectomy for transitional cell carcinoma of the bladder: results of a surgery only series in the neobladder era. J Urol 2006;176(2):486–92 [discussion: 491–2].

43. Madersbacher S, Hochreiter W, Burkhard F, et al. Radical cystectomy for bladder cancer today: a homogeneous series without neoadjuvant therapy. J Clin Oncol 2003;21(4):690–6.

44. Stein JP. Lymphadenectomy in bladder cancer: how high is "high enough"? Urol Oncol 2006;24(4): 349–55.

45. Abol-Enein H, El-Baz M, Abd El-Hameed MA, et al. Lymph node involvement in patients with bladder cancer treated with radical cystectomy: a pathoanatomical study. A single center experience. J Urol 2004;172(5 Pt 1):1818–21.

46. Vazina A, Dugi D, Shariat SF, et al. Stage specific lymph node metastasis mapping in radical cystectomy specimens. J Urol 2004;171(5):1830–4.

47. Wishnow KI, Johnson DE, Ro JY, et al. Incidence, extent and location of unsuspected pelvic lymph node metastasis in patients undergoing radical cystectomy for bladder cancer. J Urol 1987;137(3):408–10.

48. Herr HW, Bochner BH, Dalbagni G, et al. Impact of the number of lymph nodes retrieved on outcome in patients with muscle invasive bladder cancer. J Urol 2002;167(3):1295–8.

49. Dhar NB, Campbell SC, Zippe CD, et al. Outcomes in patients with urothelial carcinoma of the bladder with limited pelvic lymph node dissection. BJU Int 2006;98(6):1172–5.

50. Bochner BH, Cho D, Herr HW, et al. Prospectively packaged lymph node dissections with radical cystectomy: evaluation of node count variability and node mapping. J Urol 2004;172(4 Pt 1):1286–90.

51. Skinner DG. Management of invasive bladder cancer: a meticulous pelvic node dissection can make a difference. J Urol 1982;128(1):34–6.

52. May M, Herrmann E, Bolenz C, et al. Association between the number of dissected lymph nodes during pelvic lymphadenectomy and cancer-specific survival in patients with lymph node-negative urothelial carcinoma of the bladder undergoing radical cystectomy. Ann Surg Oncol 2011;18(7):2018–25.

53. Leissner J, Hohenfellner R, Thüroff JW, et al. Lymphadenectomy in patients with transitional cell carcinoma of the urinary bladder; significance for staging and prognosis. BJU Int 2000;85(7):817–23.

54. Koppie TM, Vickers AJ, Vora K, et al. Standardization of pelvic lymphadenectomy performed at radical cystectomy: can we establish a minimum number of lymph nodes that should be removed? Cancer 2006;107(10):2368–74.

55. Poulsen AL, Horn T, Steven K. Radical cystectomy: extending the limits of pelvic lymph node dissection improves survival for patients with bladder cancer confined to the bladder wall. J Urol 1998;160(6 Pt 1):2015–9 [discussion: 2020].

56. Abol-Enein H, Tilki D, Mosbah A, et al. Does the extent of lymphadenectomy in radical cystectomy for bladder cancer influence disease-free survival? A prospective single-center study. Eur Urol 2011; 60(3):572–7.

57. Dhar NB, Klein EA, Reuther AM, et al. Outcome after radical cystectomy with limited or extended pelvic lymph node dissection. J Urol 2008;179(3):873–8 [discussion: 878].

58. Zehnder P, Studer UE, Skinner EC, et al. Super extended versus extended pelvic lymph node dissection in patients undergoing radical cystectomy for bladder cancer: a comparative study. J Urol 2011;186(4):1261–8.

Potential Role for Targeted Therapy in Muscle-Invasive Bladder Cancer
Lessons from the Cancer Genome Atlas and Beyond

Anirban P. Mitra, MD, PhD[a], Seth P. Lerner, MD[b],*

KEYWORDS

- Urothelial carcinoma • Whole-genome sequencing • Mutation analysis • Prognosis • Clinical trials
- Targeted therapy

KEY POINTS

- Efforts of The Cancer Genome Atlas (TCGA) project and other studies have greatly advanced our understanding of genomic alterations associated with muscle-invasive bladder cancer.
- Alterations in tyrosine kinase receptors, intracellular signaling pathways, cell cycle regulators, molecular chaperones, and mediators of angiogenesis and immune response can influence bladder cancer progression and act as therapeutic targets.
- Recent whole-genome profiling studies have identified biomarker panels that can predict prognosis and may be used to identify patients who need more aggressive therapy.
- Combining surgical advances, novel targeted therapeutics, and companion theranostics represents the new paradigm for personalized treatment of muscle-invasive bladder cancer.

GENOMIC LANDSCAPE OF BLADDER CANCER

Urothelial carcinoma of the bladder (UCB) has now been recognized as evolving and progressing through at least 2 distinct molecular pathways.[1,2] Nearly 70% of low-grade noninvasive papillary tumors, which generally tend to recur locally but rarely invade and metastasize, show constitutive activation of the receptor tyrosine kinase (RTK)-Ras pathway, with activating mutations in *HRAS* and fibroblast growth factor receptor 3 (*FGFR3*) genes.[3] In contrast, carcinoma in situ (CIS) and invasive tumors show frequent alterations in the *TP53* and retinoblastoma (*RB*) genes and pathways.[4]

Although previous efforts using targeted molecular analyses have elucidated several pathways that are important for bladder tumorigenesis and cancer progression, the advent of high-throughput profiling strategies has enabled comprehensive characterization of genomic alterations for the disease.[5] Several studies have used this approach to identify genomic loci associated with the risk of developing UCB and characterizing clonal development across various disease stages.[6,7]

Disclosures: None.
[a] Department of Pathology and Center for Personalized Medicine, University of Southern California, 4650 Sunset Boulevard, SRT 1014, MS 103, Los Angeles, CA 90027, USA; [b] Translational Biology and Molecular Medicine Program, Scott Department of Urology, Dan L. Duncan Cancer Center, Baylor College of Medicine Medical Center, 7200 Cambridge, MC BCM380, A10.107, Houston, TX 77030, USA
* Corresponding author.
E-mail address: slerner@bcm.edu

Urol Clin N Am 42 (2015) 201–215
http://dx.doi.org/10.1016/j.ucl.2015.01.003
0094-0143/15/$ – see front matter © 2015 Elsevier Inc. All rights reserved.

urologic.theclinics.com

Leveraging advances in whole-genome expression profiling, next-generation sequencing, microarray analysis, and methylation arrays, The Cancer Genome Atlas (TCGA) project has comprehensively profiled 131 high-grade muscle-invasive UCBs.[8] This effort has cataloged genes that are mutated in a significant proportion of bladder cancers, several of which were not previously reported (**Table 1**). The analysis suggested that the burden of genetic alterations in UCB is similar to lung adenocarcinoma and squamous cell carcinoma and melanoma, but more than in other adult malignancies.[9]

TCGA results indicated that there were 302 exonic mutations, 204 segmental alterations in genomic copy number, and 22 genomic rearrangements on average per sample. Genes with statistically significant levels of recurrent somatic mutation were identified by Mutation Significance (MutSig) and the Catalogue of Somatic Mutations in Cancer (COSMIC) databases.[9–11] Whole exome sequencing revealed a median somatic mutation rate of 5.5 per megabase, with 49% of samples having *TP53* mutations; 12% of samples had *FGFR3* mutations that mostly affected known kinase-activating sites.

In addition to documenting genomic alterations, such efforts also have identified molecular subtypes of urothelial carcinoma. These efforts complement and extend previous studies that used pathway-based and global profiling approaches to categorize UCB based on histologic differentiation and prognosis.[12–14] Integrated mRNA, microRNA, and protein data analysis by TCGA identified 4 distinct subsets of muscle-invasive UCB.[8] A "papillary-like" cluster was enriched for tumors with papillary morphology, *FGFR3* overexpression, and associated mutations, amplifications, and translocations resulting in fusion with *TACC3* that result in constitutive activation, as previously reported by Williams and colleagues.[15] Tumors harboring these translocations may be particularly sensitive to FGFR3-targeted therapy. The remaining tumors shared genomic alterations similar to those of other tumor types, including lung adenocarcinoma, squamous cell cancers, and breast cancer. For example, 2 clusters showed features similar to luminal A breast cancer, with high expression of ERBB2 and estrogen receptor 2 (*ESR2*) signaling signature, indicating potential targets for hormone-based therapies, such as tamoxifen and raloxifene. The signature of another "basal/squamous-like" cluster resembled basal-like breast cancers and squamous cell carcinomas with overexpression of primitive cytokeratins (such as *KRT5*, *KRT6A*) and epidermal growth factor receptor (*EGFR*). First reported by Volkmer and colleagues,[13] such categorization into basal, luminal, and squamous subtypes based on molecular taxonomy also has been independently suggested by other groups.[16,17] Taken together, these observations suggest that effective targeted therapies used for other organ site cancers may provide similar benefit in patients with muscle-invasive UCB.

APPLYING GENOMICS TOWARD PROGNOSIS

Currently, clinical and histopathologic staging are the most commonly used prognostic tools for management of UCB. Statistical techniques, such as recursive partitioning and principal component analyses, have leveraged the prognostic potential of individual clinical variables to develop decision models that can predict oncological outcomes before cystectomy, thereby identifying patients who may require more aggressive therapy.[18,19] Clinical nomograms incorporate parameters such as age, gender, tumor and nodal stages, and histologic grade to estimate the risk of disease recurrence following radical cystectomy for invasive bladder cancer.[20,21] Such multivariate models can provide more accurate stratification of risk compared with single clinicopathologic prognosticators, although they are limited by the predictive power of their component clinical metrics.

Over the past 2 decades, several studies have identified individual molecular markers that are independently prognostic in UCB.[4] Such initial profiling investigations have characterized alterations in individual markers or across defined functional pathways. Several such studies concluded that a combination of markers was more prognostic than individual molecular alterations alone.[22] However, the low-to-medium throughput interrogation strategies, such as immunohistochemistry (IHC) and quantitative polymerase chain reaction, used in early investigations limited their discovery potential and were biased toward reexamining previously identified markers.[5] More recent efforts have used high-throughput unbiased approaches to interrogate coding regions of the entire genome to identify molecular panels that can distinguish disease subgroups that differ in their prognosis.[23,24] Using custom cDNA microarrays, Blaveri and colleagues[25] identified 24 unique genes based on prediction analysis that had a 78% success rate for classifying muscle-invasive bladder tumors into good and bad prognosis groups based on overall survival. Similar approaches have been used by other groups to identify multimarker gene panels that are prognostic for cancer-specific and overall survival in muscle-invasive UCB.[26–28]

Table 1
Summary of significantly mutated genes identified by The Cancer Genome Atlas project in muscle-invasive bladder cancer

Pathway/Function and Associated Gene(s)	Number of Nonsilent Mutations	Significant Association[a]
Signal transduction		
PIK3CA[b,c]	26	
FGFR3[b,c]	21	Tumor subtype[d]
ERBB3[b,c]	14	Tumor subtype[d]
ERBB2[c]	11	
TSC1[b]	11	Tumor subtype[d]
RHOB[b]	7	
HRAS[b,c]	6	
RHOA[b]	5	
CTNNB1[c]	3	
Cell cycle regulation		
TP53[b,c]	75	Tumor subtype[d]
RB1[b,c]	19	Survival
CDKN1A[b]	18	
STAG2[b]	14	
CDKN2A[b,c]	8	Disease stage
HORMAD1[b]	8	
BTG2[b]	6	
CCND3[b]	5	
Transcriptional regulation		
ELF3[b]	15	Disease stage
NFE2L2[b]	12	
RXRA[b]	12	
KLF5[b]	11	
TXNIP[b]	10	
FOXA1[b]	7	
FOXQ1[b]	7	
PAIP1[b]	7	
ZFP36L1[b]	6	
ZFR2[b]	6	
DNA damage response		
ATM[c]	19	
ERCC2[b]	16	
Histone modification/Chromatin remodeling		
ARID1A[b]	39	
MLL2[b]	39	Survival
KDM6A[b]	32	
EP300[b]	25	
Ubiquitination		
FBXW7[b,c]	16	Survival
Cell surface proteoglycan		
GPC5[b]	8	

[a] By Fisher exact test.
[b] Mutation identified by Mutation Significance (MutSig) 1.5.
[c] Mutation identified in Catalogue of Somatic Mutations in Cancer database.
[d] Papillary versus nonpapillary.

Given the prognostic value of specific molecular alterations, investigations also have examined their potential when combined with clinical nomograms. Riester and colleagues[29] reported a 20-gene signature for muscle-invasive UCB generated using Affymetrix U133 Plus 2.0 microarrays (Santa Clara, CA) that was prognostic for overall survival. When the gene signature was added to a previously reported multicenter clinical nomogram as part of a multivariate model,[20] the combined performance improved significantly over a model based on the nomogram alone. More recent studies have used whole transcriptome expression profiling to additionally interrogate noncoding RNAs that have potentially crucial regulatory roles in tumorigenesis.[30] One such study has used this approach on archival primary tumor tissues from patients with muscle-invasive UCB to identify a panel of 15 genomic features that together was prognostic for recurrence-free survival.[31] Similar to previous findings, the prognostic potential of the genomic signature was increased when combined with clinical nomograms, and the hybrid signatures outperformed nomograms by decision curve and reclassification analyses. Independent prognostic validation of such genomic signatures is crucial, given the large potential for false discovery.[32] Therefore, the previously reported genomic signature by Mitra and colleagues[31] underwent blinded independent validation in 4 external datasets, including TCGA patients, which confirmed its prognostic value. Such efforts in muscle-invasive UCB have identified reproducible prognostic biomarker panels, thereby allowing for improved and individualized patient counseling and treatment planning.

MOLECULAR TARGETING IN BLADDER CANCER

Patients with muscle-invasive UCB have a high probability of progression with regional nodal or distant visceral metastatic disease after radical cystectomy. This forebodes poor prognosis, with reported median survival less than 16 months in patients with metastatic disease.[33–36] The last drug approved for any stage of UCB was valrubicin for Bacillus Calmette-Guérin (BCG)–refractory carcinoma in 1998. There is an urgent need to introduce modern targeted therapeutics for UCB treatment, and several groups are leading the efforts to identify druggable targets. TCGA identified potential therapeutic targets in 69% of tumors, including major alterations in RTK-Ras and phosphoinositide 3-kinase/protein kinase B/mammalian target of rapamycin (PI3K/AKT/mTOR)

signaling pathways, cell cycle and transcriptional regulatory genes, and mediators of chromatin remodeling and DNA damage response (see **Table 1**). Agents targeting one or more of these pathways are in clinical trials for bladder and other malignancies.

Receptor Tyrosine Kinase Targets

Data from TCGA analysis suggest that RTK targets, such as *ERBB3* and *HRAS*, harbor recurrent mutations, whereas *ERBB2* may additionally be amplified in muscle-invasive bladder cancer (**Fig. 1**). *FGFR3* may be altered by amplification, mutation, or gene fusion. *EGFR* alterations in TCGA dataset were entirely due to gene amplification. Indeed, EGFR overexpression is noted in nearly three-fourths of all UCBs, which make them attractive targets for monoclonal antibodies (cetuximab, panitumumab) and oral RTK inhibitors (erlotinib, gefitinib).[37] However, phase II trials of cetuximab in the setting of metastatic UCB have yielded mixed results.[38,39] Results for gefitinib as a single agent or in combination with chemotherapy for metastatic UCB also have been disappointing.[40,41] Nevertheless, erlotinib has shown some activity in the neoadjuvant setting with a trial of 20 patients with cT2 UCB treated before cystectomy showing a 25% downstaging rate to pT0.[42] It is currently the subject of 2 ongoing phase II trials (ClinicalTrials.gov, NCT00749892 and NCT00380029) (**Box 1**).

Analysis of the COSMIC database revealed that *ERBB2* was a significantly mutated gene in muscle-invasive UCBs.[8] Trastuzumab, a monoclonal antibody that targets the HER2 protein encoded by *ERBB2*, is efficacious in breast and gastroesophageal cancers that overexpress the marker.[43,44] Initial results of a phase I/II trial in patients with muscle-invasive UCB with HER2 overexpressing (2+ or 3+ by IHC) tumors undergoing definitive therapy with concurrent radiation, paclitaxel, and trastuzumab following transurethral surgery who were not candidates for cystectomy (ClinicalTrials.gov, NCT00238420) suggested that trimodality bladder-preserving therapy may be appropriate for such candidates with invasive UCB.[45] Complete response rate was 69% in patients receiving trastuzumab compared with 58% in those who did not, although adverse events, including bone marrow suppression, were higher in the former group.

DN24-02, an autologous cellular immunotherapeutic that is manufactured using the same platform as sipuleucel-T, targets HER2-expressing UCB cells. NEU Active Cellular immunotherapy (NeuACT) is an ongoing phase II trial that

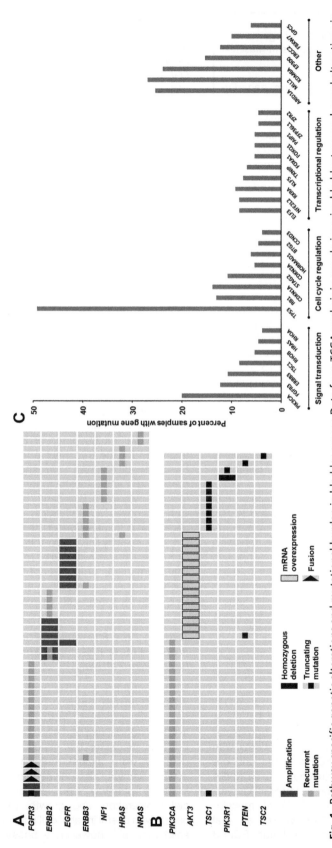

Fig. 1. Pathway-specific genetic alterations and mutational burden in bladder cancer. Data from TCGA analysis in muscle-invasive bladder tumors showed alterations in (A) RTKs by amplification, mutation, or fusion, and (B) PI3K/AKT/mTOR pathway that are mutually exclusive. Tumor samples are shown in columns and genes in rows; only samples with at least one alteration are shown. (C) Genes with statistically significant levels of mutation as detected by MutSig across normal-bladder tumor pairs. (*Adapted from* The Cancer Genome Atlas Research Network. Comprehensive molecular characterization of urothelial bladder carcinoma. Nature 2014;507(7492):319; with permission.)

randomizes patients with HER2 overexpressing UCBs (1+, 2+, or 3+ by IHC) to adjuvant DN24-02 or observation after radical cystectomy (ClinicalTrials.gov, NCT01353222) (see **Box 1**). Early results indicate that more than 75% of patients have HER2 overexpression ($\geq$1+) in primary tumors and positive lymph nodes.[46] Data also suggested an immunologic prime-boost effect and prolonged humoral immune responses with DN24-02. These studies also illustrate the variable criteria regarding what represents HER2-positivity in UCB for optimal patient selection for treatment with HER2-targeting agents.

Lapatinib, an oral bifunctional RTK inhibitor, has been used for dual targeting of EGFR and HER2. In the setting of second-line therapy in patients with locally advanced or metastatic UCB, it showed little activity in unselected patients (objective response, 1.7%; stable disease, 31%).[47] However, further analysis demonstrated an improvement in overall survival in a subset of patients with tumors overexpressing EGFR and/or HER2. It was being studied in the neoadjuvant setting as a phase 0 trial for patients with muscle-invasive UCB who were candidates for cystectomy, but was prematurely terminated because of poor enrollment (Clinical Trials.gov, NCT01245660).

Although activating point mutations of *FGFR3* are more common in noninvasive UCB, TCGA analysis noted such mutations in 12% of muscle-invasive tumors (see **Fig. 1**).[8,48] In patients with advanced-stage tumors, *FGFR3* mutations are more frequently seen in conjunction with *CDKN2A* deletion.[49] Other studies have noted FGFR3 over-expression in approximately 50% of muscle-invasive bladder cancers.[50] Dovitinib, an oral multitargeted RTK inhibitor that binds FGFR3

among others, has been tested in a phase II trial in advanced UCB.[51] The study was terminated when it was determined that there was limited single-agent activity in patients regardless of their *FGFR3* mutation status. Nevertheless, a phase II trial of dovitinib in patients with BCG-refractory non–muscle-invasive UCBs with *FGFR3* mutations or overexpression is currently under way (Clinical Trials.gov, NCT01732107). Phase I trials with novel pan-FGFR inhibitors, such as JNJ-42756493 and BGJ398, also suggest activity in patients with tumors harboring *FGFR3*-activating mutations and *FGFR3-TACC3* translocations.[52,53]

Sunitinib is a multitargeted RTK inhibitor that is approved for the treatment of renal cell carcinoma and imatinib-resistant gastrointestinal stromal tumors.[54] Preclinical studies have shown that it enhances the activity of cisplatin against UCB, possibly by targeting the stroma.[55] A single-agent phase II study showed modest responses in the setting of metastatic UCB, although it failed to reach the predetermined threshold for antitumor activity.[56] Final results are awaited on a phase II single-arm trial evaluating the combination of sunitinib with gemcitabine and cisplatin as neoadjuvant therapy in patients with muscle-invasive UCB (ClinicalTrials.gov, NCT00847015), although a smaller trial reported excessive toxicity with the combination of these drugs in this setting.[57] Dasatinib is another oral multitargeted RTK inhibitor that is approved for the treatment of certain leukemias. Dasatinib administration was shown to be feasible preceding radical cystectomy in patients with muscle-invasive UCB as part of a phase II trial (ClinicalTrials.gov, NCT00706641), with a marked decrease in expression of phosphorylated SRC family kinases by IHC in two-thirds of all cases.[58,59] Correlative studies with a view to identifying molecular biomarkers predictive of response will be needed if a subset of patients is to benefit from RTK-targeted therapeutics in the future.

Targeting the Phosphoinositide 3-Kinase/Protein Kinase B/Mammalian Target of Rapamycin Pathway

More than 40% of UCBs have alterations in the PI3K/AKT/mTOR pathway.[60] TCGA reports the mutational burden of *PIK3CA* and *TSC1* in UCBs at 20% and 8%, respectively (see **Fig. 1**). The analysis also suggested that genetic alterations in this pathway were almost mutually exclusive. The mTOR pathway is downstream of the PI3K signaling pathway, and regulates metabolism, cell proliferation, and growth. mTOR inhibition has proven useful in renal cell carcinoma and other solid tumors[61]; however, a phase II trial of the mTOR inhibitor everolimus in locally advanced UCB showed disappointing results with partial response seen in 2 of 37 evaluable patients.[62] Another single-arm phase II study investigating everolimus in 45 patients with metastatic UCB reported 1 partial response, 1 near-complete response, and 12 minor regressions.[63] Whole-genome sequencing of the tumor of a patient who achieved durable (>2 years) everolimus response showed a loss-of-function mutation in TSC1.[64] Analysis of 13 additional patients with UCB treated on the same trial by targeted deep sequencing revealed 3 additional tumors harboring inactivating TSC1 mutations, including 2 patients who had minor responses to everolimus, thereby suggesting this mutation as a possible biomarker of therapeutic response. In contrast, tumors from 8 of the 9 patients showing disease progression were TSC1 wild type. Oral everolimus is currently being investigated in a phase I/II trial in combination with intravesical gemcitabine for BCG-refractory CIS of the bladder (ClinicalTrials.gov, NCT01259063).

Cell Cycle Targets

Invasive UCBs classically have been associated with loss of cell cycle control.[65] TP53 mutation is the most common genetic alteration in muscle-invasive UCBs (see Fig. 1). TCGA analysis also revealed that TP53 mutations were mutually exclusive in their relationship with overexpression and amplification of MDM2, thereby resulting in inactivation of p53 function in 76% of samples.[8] Alterations in p53 and its associated proteins may be prognostic in bladder cancer.[22,66–68] However, although early reports suggested that p53 expression may be prognostic in organ-confined muscle-invasive UCB,[69] this was not confirmed in the prospective setting.[70]

Defects in the RB pathway are another major mechanism by which cell cycle control is lost in UCB.[71] This can occur through inactivating RB mutations, RB hyperphosphorylation, and/or alterations in cyclins, p16, and/or E2Fs.[72] RB1 mutations were noted in 13% of TCGA samples, although significant mutations also were noted in CDKN1A, CDKN2A, and CCND3 (see Fig. 1). Alterations in the RB pathway also may be prognostic in UCB.[73–75]

The cyclin-dependent kinase 4/6 (CDK 4/6) complex combines with cyclin D1 to inhibit RB activity.[76] Therapeutic targeting of this complex with palbociclib improves outcome in estrogen receptor-positive advanced breast cancer. A randomized phase II trial of 165 women in this setting reported a median progression-free survival of 10.2 months in patients treated with letrozole alone compared with 20.2 months in patients treated with letrozole

and palbociclib.[77] This combination is now being tested in a confirmatory phase III trial in this setting (ClinicalTrials.gov, NCT01740427). A phase II trial of palbociclib is currently being planned in patients with metastatic UCB who have progressed after first-line chemotherapy (ClinicalTrials.gov, NCT02334527). Manipulation of RB and other cell cycle regulatory pathways thus represents a highly attractive set of targets given their frequency of oncogenic alterations in UCB.

Angiogenesis Targets

Angiogenesis involves interaction of tumor cell–derived factors with stromal elements to recruit endothelial cells to the site of malignancy and establish a vascular supply, which provides nutrients for rapid clonal expansion of the cancer cells. Angiogenesis, as measured histologically by microvessel density estimations, can predict UCB outcomes.[78] Overexpression of angiogenic mediators, including hypoxia-inducible factors, vascular endothelial growth factor (VEGF), and basic fibroblast growth factor, have been correlated with poor prognosis in UCB.[2] Alterations in expression of VEGF receptors, such as VEGFR2, also have been implicated in promoting tumor invasion and nodal metastasis.[79,80] A greater understanding of the central role of angiogenesis in UCB progression, and the availability of antiangiogenic agents has prompted their evaluation in bladder cancer.

The combination of bevacizumab, an anti-VEGF monoclonal antibody, with chemotherapy has been assessed in a phase II trial as a first-line treatment in metastatic UCB.[81] Gemcitabine and cisplatin were combined with bevacizumab in 43 patients, resulting in an overall response rate of 72% and an overall survival of 19.1 months. This regimen is now being tested in a randomized phase III trial comparing gemcitabine and cisplatin with or without bevacizumab in patients with locally advanced or metastatic UCB (ClinicalTrials.gov, NCT00942331). This trial has completed accrual and results are pending. The combination of bevacizumab with methotrexate, vinblastine, adriamycin and cisplatin (MVAC) administered as dose-dense therapy has also been examined as part of a phase II trial in the neoadjuvant setting for high-risk urothelial cancer.[82] In this study, pathological downstaging to ≤pT1N0M0 was observed in 45% of patients with UCB. Final results also are awaited on a phase II trial evaluating aflibercept, a VEGF inhibitor, for patients with recurrent, locally advanced, or metastatic UCB (ClinicalTrials.gov, NCT00407485).

Sorafenib, which inhibits a number of targets, including VEGF, has been tested as a monotherapy for advanced-stage UCB in phase II trials. However, the drug failed to show any objective responses in first-line and second-line settings.[83,84] Sunitinib, another multitargeted RTK inhibitor that also inhibits VEGF, is being assessed as neoadjuvant therapy in patients with muscle-invasive UCB, as noted previously. Vandetanib, an oral inhibitor of VGFR2 and EGFR, did not result in a significant improvement in response rate or survival when added to docetaxel as part of a phase II trial of 142 patients with metastatic UCB who progressed on previous platinum-based chemotherapy.[85] Pazopanib, a VEGFR-targeted RTK inhibitor, has demonstrated partial response in 17% of the 41 patients in a phase II study of chemorefractory advanced-stage UCB.[86] Although several of these small molecular inhibitors have yet to be tested for clinically localized muscle-invasive UCB, their modest activity in patients with metastatic disease suggests that more optimal patient selection is required before further assessment is made for localized disease.

Stress Response Targets

Heat shock proteins (HSP) act as molecular chaperones to stabilize signaling proteins, and are upregulated during cellular stress.[87] HSP27 is an ATP-independent cytoprotective chaperone with well-described tumorigenic and metastatic roles.[88] It mediates malignant progression of cancer cells through increased tumorigenicity, treatment resistance, and inhibition of apoptosis. HSP27 overexpression can result in activation of AKT, thereby leading to extracellular signal-regulated kinase translocation to the nucleus and increased cell proliferation.[89] HSP27 is overexpressed in UCBs and has been implicated in chemoresistance.[90] Intravesical instillation of OGX-427, a second-generation antisense oligonucleotide that targets HSP27 mRNA, has shown antitumor activity with minimal toxicity in an orthotopic mouse model of high-grade UCB.[91] It is being tested in 2 randomized phase II trials in patients with inoperable advanced UCB. The first trial is comparing the value of gemcitabine-cisplatin chemotherapy with or without OGX-427 (Clinical Trials.gov, NCT01454089), and the second trial is examining docetaxel with or without OGX-427 in the second-line setting in patients with relapsed or refractory metastatic UCB (ClinicalTrials.gov, NCT01780545). Early reports from the first trial indicate that addition of 600 mg OGX-427 to gemcitabine-cisplatin chemotherapy showed a 14% reduction in overall mortality and 17% reduction in disease progression when compared with chemotherapy alone.[92] Patients with lower performance status derived the greatest benefit, resulting in a 50% reduction in overall mortality compared with chemotherapy alone. This has led to plans to test OGX-427 (600 mg and maintenance) in the setting of a phase III trial. If OGX-427 is conclusively shown to improve the efficacy of cytotoxic chemotherapy in metastatic disease, conducting similar investigations for muscle-invasive UCB would be warranted.

Targeting the Immune System

Immunotherapy has been used as a proven treatment paradigm for patients with prostate and renal cancers for several years. Although multiple antigenic targets have been identified, vaccine development is still in its early stages in UCB. Only safety data for vaccination are available thus far and their efficacy remains to be demonstrated.[93,94] Anti–CTLA-4 (cytotoxic T lymphocyte antigen-4) antibodies are thought to inhibit development of tolerance to tumor cells by the immune system.[95] These antibodies have been studied in the neoadjuvant setting, but only safety data are available.[96] Monoclonal antibodies targeting CTLA-4 include ipilimumab and tremelimumab. A single-arm phase II trial assessing the efficacy of first-line gemcitabine-cisplatin with ipilimumab for metastatic UCB is currently under way (ClinicalTrials.gov, NCT01524991).

Programmed death-ligand 1 (PD-L1) is a protein that is thought to suppress the immune system during normal events, such as pregnancy, but may be upregulated in cancers thereby allowing them to evade the host immune system.[97] Blockade of the interaction between PD-L1 and its receptor by anti–PD-L1 antibodies have been shown to potentiate immune responses and mediate antitumor activity.[98] The receptor for PD-L1 may be blocked by monoclonal antibodies including pembrolizumab, nivolumab, and AMP-514, and these have been tested in various cancers. PD-L1 itself may be targeted by human monoclonal antibodies, such as MPDL3280A and MEDI4736. MPDL3280A is an anti–PD-L1 immunotherapeutic that was well tolerated in a phase I expansion study with an adaptive design in patients with previously treated metastatic UCB.[99] At a minimum follow-up of 6 weeks, objective responses were noted in 43% of patients with positive PD-L1 expression in tumor-infiltrating immune cells (IHC 2+ or 3+) and 11% of those with negative PD-L1 expression (IHC 0 or 1+). This has led to a phase II single-arm study of MPDL3280A in patients with locally advanced or metastatic UCB (ClinicalTrials.gov, NCT02108652). Another ongoing large phase III randomized study is comparing MPDL3280A with chemotherapy in a similar group of patients after failing platinum-based regimens (ClinicalTrials.gov, NCT023 02807). Results of these trials are awaited.

The previously discussed examples highlight the wide range of targeted agents being tested, alone or in combination with cytotoxic drugs, in clinical trials for UCB. These agents have the potential to provide promising new therapeutic options for patients with this disease.

PREDICTORS OF THERAPEUTIC RESPONSE

It follows from the preceding discussion that there are a number of molecular alterations in bladder cancer, several of which can be targeting by novel therapeutics. However, not all trials of such agents have posted remarkable results, which suggest the need for more accurate identification of patient subpopulations that stand to derive the most benefit from specific therapies. This has led to the growth of companion diagnostics and thera-nostics for specific molecular alterations.[100] Such streamlined approaches can result in more accurate patient selection, thereby increasing the likelihood of achieving maximal oncologic response in patients who are the most ideal candidates to benefit from targeted agents.

Combination chemotherapy that contains DNA-damaging agents, such as cisplatin, currently remains the established standard for muscle-invasive UCB, improving overall survival as established by prospective studies.[101] The addition of neoadjuvant chemotherapy to radical cystectomy has been shown to increase disease-free survival by 9% in this setting.[102] Therefore, identification of molecular alterations that render UCB sensitive to cisplatin-containing regimens could potentially allow chemotherapy to be restricted to those who derive maximal benefit, thereby sparing more than 90% of patients unnecessary toxicity. The concept of identifying patients who may respond the best to anticancer therapies was tested even before the advent of targeted agents for UCB treatment. Early evidence suggested that patients with locally advanced UCB who harbor p53 alterations beneficially respond to cisplatin-containing adjuvant chemotherapy regimens.[103] The plausible explanation was that DNA damage to p53-altered urothelial cells may cause an "uncoupling" of the S and M phases of the cell cycle, thereby resulting in apoptosis.[104] This was the basis for an international multicenter phase III trial for patients with organ-confined UCB who were randomized to adjuvant therapy with MVAC versus observation if their primary tumors demonstrated altered p53 status as assessed by IHC.[70] The underlying hypothesis was that p53 alteration in the primary tumor is associated with worse prognosis, and these patients also would benefit from adjuvant cisplatin-containing chemotherapy. The trial was closed before reaching its full accrual target after a planned interim analysis suggested that the probability of detecting a significant difference in time to recurrence in the randomized population would be highly unlikely. The trial also did not demonstrate prognostic value of p53 IHC in large part because of the overall favorable outcome of the cohort, which was markedly better than the cohort described by Esrig and colleagues.[69] Secondary analyses comparing p53 protein alterations as determined by IHC with *TP53* genotypic alterations to determine the role of exonic mutations with progression and chemotherapeutic response is currently ongoing. Although the results were negative, this was the first trial in urologic cancers that used a predictive biomarker to select therapy and serves as a model for future UCB studies that incorporate molecular diagnostics.[105]

More recently, Als and colleagues[106] identified a 55-gene signature that was predictive for survival following cisplatin-based chemotherapy for locally advanced or metastatic UCB. Emmprin and survivin were shortlisted for further validation by IHC, which were found to be significantly correlated with progression-free, disease-specific, and overall survival. In patients without visceral metastases, those with 0, 1+, and 2+ IHC scores had estimated 5-year survival rates of 44.0%, 21.1%, and 0%, respectively. In the setting of neoadjuvant MVAC chemotherapy, Takata and colleagues[107] used high-throughput expression profiling to identify a 14-gene signature that had a 100% negative predictive value for downstaging muscle-invasive UCB to ≤T1 disease. Further validation using additional cases confirmed the accuracy, sensitivity, and specificity of the signature at 92.5%, 100.0%, and 72.7%, respectively.[108] The same group later developed another 12-gene signature to predict response to gemcitabine-carboplatin neoadjuvant chemotherapy, which accurately predicted drug responses in 18 of 19 test cases.[109] The findings have led to an ongoing prospective study that aims to validate these predictive gene signatures.[110] Other studies also have indicated roles for other individual biomarkers predictive of response to platinum-based chemotherapy, including excision repair cross-complementation group 1 (*ERCC1*), multidrug resistance gene 1 (*MDR1*), and breast cancer susceptibility gene 1 (*BRCA1*).[111–113]

Another strategy to derive predictive biomarker panels uses expression results derived from in vitro cell line screens in a coexpression extrapolation (COXEN) algorithm to identify drug sensitivity signatures.[114] This approach has been used to accurately predict drug sensitivity of bladder cancer cell lines and clinical outcomes of patients with UCB undergoing systemic MVAC therapy.[115] The predictive ability of the COXEN score is now being investigated prospectively in a phase II trial that randomizes patients with muscle-invasive UCB to neoadjuvant gemcitabine-cisplatin or dose-dense MVAC (ClinicalTrials.gov, NCT0217 7695). The primary end point of this trial is to determine whether the treatment-specific COXEN score is predictive of 3-month complete response to neoadjuvant chemotherapy. If the trial is positive, a subsequent trial will use the COXEN score to direct therapy between the 2 neoadjuvant chemotherapy regimens.

Given the advances in "omic" technologies and knowledge derived from TCGA studies, the National Cancer Institute is set to launch a series of clinical studies with the overall aim of using more precise diagnostics to direct patient selection for therapies that target particular molecular abnormalities.[116] The Molecular Analysis for Therapy Choice (MATCH) program is a prospective clinical trial that will assign treatment hypothesized to target selected molecular abnormalities based on a tumor's molecular profile. MATCH will include several small trials for patients with metastatic tumors that are no longer responding to standard therapy. Specifically, it will feature an umbrella protocol for multiple, single-arm phase II trials with each molecular patient subgroup matched to a targeted agent. Patients whose cancers progress during the first assigned treatment may be able to go on to another MATCH trial arm if they have a second actionable molecular target in their tumors. In addition, any patient whose cancer initially shrinks and then progresses during the trial will be eligible to have their tumors reprofiled and, if they have a genetic change that is targeted by another drug being tested in MATCH, they may be eligible to enroll in one of the other phase II MATCH trials. This paradigm will likely also be implemented in patients with metastatic UCB in whom frontline therapy has failed. Currently, it is proposed that actionable targets in UCB for this trial will include alterations in *FGFR3*, the PI3K/AKT/mTOR pathway, and RB inactivation.

Several alternative strategies have been used in other malignancies to leverage the information derived from genomic analyses of patient tumors to drive therapeutic management. The S1400 Lung Master Protocol (Lung-MAP), sponsored by the Southwest Oncology Group, is one such example that uses biomarker-targeted therapy to treat patients with advanced lung cancer (Clinical Trials.gov, NCT02154490). Lung-MAP is a large-scale, phase II/III trial that will assess genomes of patients with recurrent stage IIIB-IV squamous cell lung cancer moving to second-line therapy to direct them to the most appropriate substudy. Each substudy is designed around a genomically defined alteration in the tumor and a corresponding targeted therapeutic. Patients on each substudy are randomized to either standard of care (docetaxel or erlotinib) or biomarker-driven targeted therapy with an investigational agent. Each substudy functions autonomously, opens and closes independently, and is independently powered for overall survival with an interim analysis for progression-free survival to determine whether to proceed from phase II to phase III. When a substudy end point is met, the drug-biomarker combination may proceed for regulatory approval review. When an end point is not met, the substudy will be closed and another modular substudy of a different agent will be initiated. If Lung-MAP is successful, it could serve as a prototype for drug registration in other settings.

The National Cancer Institute has also recently implemented the Exceptional Responders Initiative, a study that investigates the molecular factors associated with exceptional responses to anticancer drug therapies (ClinicalTrials.gov, NCT022 43592). This initiative will attempt to identify molecular features in tumors that predict whether a particular drug or drug class will be beneficial. Tumor specimens from patients in clinical trials who achieved an exceptional response relative to other trial participants, or other patients who achieved an exceptional and unexpected response to a noninvestigational therapy will be profiled to identify predictive markers. Discovery of such molecular markers may allow for more effective selection of treatment programs, thereby identifying individual patients who may potentially respond to agents with the same or similar mechanism of action. Implementation of such precision medicine trials in the realm of UCB is the ultimate goal of personalized medicine.

SUMMARY

Bladder cancer is a disease with a complex molecular mechanism of tumorigenesis and progression that can pose challenges for conventional therapeutic approaches. There is a clear need for improved systemic therapies for treatment of muscle-invasive UCB, as approximately 50% of patients will relapse and die from distant metastases after local therapy.[117] Advances in understanding of the molecular biology behind this disease and advent of novel targeted therapeutics can play a dual role in better outcome prediction and more effective treatment regimens.

Integrated molecular analytical efforts including those from TCGA have identified several actionable genetic alterations that may be useful for personalizing therapeutic strategies. However, there are still several unmet needs for translating these findings and implementing targeted therapies, including (1) access to affordable and clinical-grade sequencing platforms, (2) companion diagnostics to identify drug targets, (3) validated assays that can predict therapeutic responses, (4) targeted agents tested in early-phase studies for UCB, and (5) addressing regulatory and funding challenges for implementing targeted therapy trials.[118] Despite these challenges, breakthroughs in genomic data mining, improved mechanistic understanding of drug resistance, and accelerated progress in development and testing of novel therapeutics in muscle-invasive UCB are paving the way for a more individualized and effective approach to cancer treatment.

REFERENCES

1. Spruck CH III, Ohneseit PF, Gonzalez-Zulueta M, et al. Two molecular pathways to transitional cell carcinoma of the bladder. Cancer Res 1994; 54(3):784–8.

2. Mitra AP, Cote RJ. Molecular pathogenesis and diagnostics of bladder cancer. Annu Rev Pathol 2009;4:251–85.

3. Pasin E, Josephson DY, Mitra AP, et al. Superficial bladder cancer: an update on etiology, molecular development, classification, and natural history. Rev Urol 2008;10(1):31–43.

4. Mitra AP, Datar RH, Cote RJ. Molecular pathways in invasive bladder cancer: new insights into mechanisms, progression, and target identification. J Clin Oncol 2006;24(35):5552–64.

5. Mitra AP, Bartsch CC, Cote RJ. Strategies for molecular expression profiling in bladder cancer. Cancer Metastasis Rev 2009;28(3–4):317–26.

6. Figueroa JD, Ye Y, Siddiq A, et al. Genome-wide association study identifies multiple loci associated with bladder cancer risk. Hum Mol Genet 2014; 23(5):1387–98.

7. Nordentoft I, Lamy P, Birkenkamp-Demtröder K, et al. Mutational context and diverse clonal development in early and late bladder cancer. Cell Rep 2014;7(5):1649–63.

8. The Cancer Genome Atlas Research Network. Comprehensive molecular characterization of urothelial bladder carcinoma. Nature 2014;507(7492): 315–22.

9. Lawrence MS, Stojanov P, Polak P, et al. Mutational heterogeneity in cancer and the search for new cancer-associated genes. Nature 2013;499(7457): 214–8.

10. Lawrence MS, Stojanov P, Mermel CH, et al. Discovery and saturation analysis of cancer genes across 21 tumour types. Nature 2014;505(7484): 495–501.

11. Forbes SA, Bindal N, Bamford S, et al. COSMIC: mining complete cancer genomes in the Catalogue of Somatic Mutations in Cancer. Nucleic Acids Res 2011;39(Database Issue):D945–50.

12. Dyrskjøt L, Thykjaer T, Kruhoffer M, et al. Identifying distinct classes of bladder carcinoma using microarrays. Nat Genet 2003;33(1):90–6.

13. Volkmer JP, Sahoo D, Chin RK, et al. Three differentiation states risk-stratify bladder cancer into distinct subtypes. Proc Natl Acad Sci U S A 2012;109(6):2078–83.

14. Mitra AP, Pagliarulo V, Yang D, et al. Generation of a concise gene panel for outcome prediction in urinary bladder cancer. J Clin Oncol 2009;27(24): 3929–37.

15. Williams SV, Hurst CD, Knowles MA. Oncogenic FGFR3 gene fusions in bladder cancer. Hum Mol Genet 2013;22(4):795–803.

16. Sjödahl G, Lauss M, Lövgren K, et al. A molecular taxonomy for urothelial carcinoma. Clin Cancer Res 2012;18(12):3377–86.

17. Choi W, Porten S, Kim S, et al. Identification of distinct basal and luminal subtypes of muscle-invasive bladder cancer with different sensitivities to frontline chemotherapy. Cancer Cell 2014;25(2):152–65.

18. Mitra AP, Skinner EC, Miranda G, et al. A precystectomy decision model to predict pathological upstaging and oncological outcomes in clinical stage T2 bladder cancer. BJU Int 2013; 111(2):240–8.

19. Ahmadi H, Mitra AP, Abdelsayed GA, et al. Principal component analysis based pre-cystectomy model to predict pathological stage in patients with clinical organ-confined bladder cancer. BJU Int 2013;111(4 Pt B):E167–72.

20. International Bladder Cancer Nomogram Consortium. Postoperative nomogram predicting risk of recurrence after radical cystectomy for bladder cancer. J Clin Oncol 2006;24(24):3967–72.

21. Shariat SF, Karakiewicz PI, Palapattu GS, et al. Nomograms provide improved accuracy for predicting survival after radical cystectomy. Clin Cancer Res 2006;12(22):6663–76.

22. Birkhahn M, Mitra AP, Cote RJ. Molecular markers for bladder cancer: the road to a multimarker approach. Expert Rev Anticancer Ther 2007; 7(12):1717–27.

23. Dyrskjøt L, Zieger K, Kruhoffer M, et al. A molecular signature in superficial bladder carcinoma predicts

clinical outcome. Clin Cancer Res 2005;11(11): 4029–36.

24. Wild PJ, Herr A, Wissmann C, et al. Gene expression profiling of progressive papillary noninvasive carcinomas of the urinary bladder. Clin Cancer Res 2005;11(12):4415–29.

25. Blaveri E, Simko JP, Korkola JE, et al. Bladder cancer outcome and subtype classification by gene expression. Clin Cancer Res 2005;11(11):4044–55.

26. Sanchez-Carbayo M, Socci ND, Lozano J, et al. Defining molecular profiles of poor outcome in patients with invasive bladder cancer using oligonucleotide microarrays. J Clin Oncol 2006;24(5): 778–89.

27. Kim WJ, Kim EJ, Kim SK, et al. Predictive value of progression-related gene classifier in primary non-muscle invasive bladder cancer. Mol Cancer 2010; 9:3.

28. Kim WJ, Kim SK, Jeong P, et al. A four-gene signature predicts disease progression in muscle invasive bladder cancer. Mol Med 2011;17(5–6): 478–85.

29. Riester M, Taylor JM, Feifer A, et al. Combination of a novel gene expression signature with a clinical nomogram improves the prediction of survival in high-risk bladder cancer. Clin Cancer Res 2012; 18(5):1323–33.

30. Mitra SA, Mitra AP, Triche TJ. A central role for long non-coding RNA in cancer. Front Genet 2012;3:17.

31. Mitra AP, Lam LL, Ghadessi M, et al. Discovery and validation of novel expression signature for post-cystectomy recurrence in high-risk bladder cancer. J Natl Cancer Inst 2014;106(11). pii:dju290.

32. Dyrskjøt L, Zieger K, Real FX, et al. Gene expression signatures predict outcome in non-muscle-invasive bladder carcinoma: a multicenter validation study. Clin Cancer Res 2007;13(12): 3545–51.

33. Bellmunt J, von der Maase H, Mead GM, et al. Randomized phase III study comparing paclitaxel/cisplatin/gemcitabine and gemcitabine/cisplatin in patients with locally advanced or metastatic urothelial cancer without prior systemic therapy: EORTC Intergroup Study 30987. J Clin Oncol 2012;30(10):1107–13.

34. von der Maase H, Sengelov L, Roberts JT, et al. Long-term survival results of a randomized trial comparing gemcitabine plus cisplatin, with methotrexate, vinblastine, doxorubicin, plus cisplatin in patients with bladder cancer. J Clin Oncol 2005; 23(21):4602–8.

35. Rink M, Lee DJ, Kent M, et al. Predictors of cancer-specific mortality after disease recurrence following radical cystectomy. BJU Int 2013;111(3 Pt B): E30–6.

36. Mitra AP, Quinn DI, Dorff TB, et al. Factors influencing post-recurrence survival in bladder cancer

following radical cystectomy. BJU Int 2012;109(6): 846–54.

37. Chaux A, Cohen JS, Schultz L, et al. High epidermal growth factor receptor immunohistochemical expression in urothelial carcinoma of the bladder is not associated with EGFR mutations in exons 19 and 21: a study using formalin-fixed, paraffin-embedded archival tissues. Hum Pathol 2012;43(10):1590–5.

38. Wong YN, Litwin S, Vaughn D, et al. Phase II trial of cetuximab with or without paclitaxel in patients with advanced urothelial tract carcinoma. J Clin Oncol 2012;30(28):3545–51.

39. Hussain M, Daignault S, Agarwal N, et al. A randomized phase 2 trial of gemcitabine/cisplatin with or without cetuximab in patients with advanced urothelial carcinoma. Cancer 2014; 120(17):2684–93.

40. Petrylak DP, Tangen CM, Van Veldhuizen PJ Jr, et al. Results of the Southwest Oncology Group phase II evaluation (study S0031) of ZD1839 for advanced transitional cell carcinoma of the urothelium. BJU Int 2010;105(3):317–21.

41. Philips GK, Halabi S, Sanford BL, et al. A phase II trial of cisplatin (C), gemcitabine (G) and gefitinib for advanced urothelial tract carcinoma: results of cancer and leukemia group B (CALGB) 90102. Ann Oncol 2009;20(6):1074–9.

42. Pruthi RS, Nielsen M, Heathcote S, et al. A phase II trial of neoadjuvant erlotinib in patients with muscle-invasive bladder cancer undergoing radical cystectomy: clinical and pathological results. BJU Int 2010;106(3):349–54.

43. Moja L, Tagliabue L, Balduzzi S, et al. Trastuzumab containing regimens for early breast cancer. Cochrane Database Syst Rev 2012;(4):CD006243.

44. Bang YJ, Van Cutsem E, Feyereislova A, et al. Trastuzumab in combination with chemotherapy versus chemotherapy alone for treatment of HER2-positive advanced gastric or gastro-oesophageal junction cancer (ToGA): a phase 3, open-label, randomised controlled trial. Lancet 2010;376(9742):687–97.

45. Michaelson MD, Hu C, Pham HT, et al. The initial report of RTOG 0524: phase I/II trial of a combination of paclitaxel and trastuzumab with daily irradiation or paclitaxel alone with daily irradiation following transurethral surgery for noncystectomy candidates with muscle-invasive bladder cancer. J Clin Oncol 2014;32(Suppl 4):LBA287.

46. Bajorin DF, Sharma P, Gomella LG, et al. NeuACT, a phase II, randomized, open-label trial of DN24-02: updated analysis of HER2 expression, immune responses, product parameters, and safety in patients with surgically resected HER2+ urothelial cancer. J Clin Oncol 2014;32(Suppl 4):296.

47. Wülfing C, Machiels JP, Richel DJ, et al. A single-arm, multicenter, open-label phase 2 study of

lapatinib as the second-line treatment of patients with locally advanced or metastatic transitional cell carcinoma. Cancer 2009;115(13):2881–90.

48. Bartsch G, Mitra AP, Cote RJ. Expression profiling for bladder cancer: strategies to uncover prognostic factors. Expert Rev Anticancer Ther 2010; 10(12):1945–54.

49. Rebouissou S, Herault A, Letouze E, et al. CDKN2A homozygous deletion is associated with muscle invasion in FGFR3-mutated urothelial bladder carcinoma. J Pathol 2012;227(3):315–24.

50. Tomlinson DC, Baldo O, Harnden P, et al. FGFR3 protein expression and its relationship to mutation status and prognostic variables in bladder cancer. J Pathol 2007;213(1):91–8.

51. Milowsky MI, Dittrich C, Durán I, et al. Phase 2 trial of dovitinib in patients with progressive FGFR3-mutated or FGFR3 wild-type advanced urothelial carcinoma. Eur J Cancer 2014;50(18):3145–52.

52. Bahleda R, Dienstmann R, Adamo B, et al. Phase 1 study of JNJ-42756493, a pan-fibroblast growth factor receptor (FGFR) inhibitor, in patients with advanced solid tumors. J Clin Oncol 2014; 32(Suppl 5):2501.

53. Sequist LV, Cassier P, Varga A, et al. Phase I study of BGJ398, a selective pan-FGFR inhibitor in genetically preselected advanced solid tumors. Cancer Res 2014;74(Suppl 19):CT326.

54. Youssef RF, Mitra AP, Bartsch G Jr, et al. Molecular targets and targeted therapies in bladder cancer management. World J Urol 2009;27(1):9–20.

55. Sonpavde G, Jian W, Liu H, et al. Sunitinib malate is active against human urothelial carcinoma and enhances the activity of cisplatin in a preclinical model. Urol Oncol 2009;27(4):391–9.

56. Gallagher DJ, Milowsky MI, Gerst SR, et al. Phase II study of sunitinib in patients with metastatic urothelial cancer. J Clin Oncol 2010;28(8):1373–9.

57. Galsky MD, Hahn NM, Powles T, et al. Gemcitabine, cisplatin, and sunitinib for metastatic urothelial carcinoma and as preoperative therapy for muscle-invasive bladder cancer. Clin Genitourin Cancer 2013;11(2):175–81.

58. Hahn NM, Daneshmand S, Posadas EM, et al. A phase II trial of neoadjuvant dasatinib (Neo-D) in muscle-invasive urothelial carcinoma of the bladder (miUCB): Hoosier Oncology Group GU07–122 trial. J Clin Oncol 2012;30(Suppl 15):4586.

59. Knudsen B, Hahn NM, Daneshmand S, et al. Biologic activity of dasatinib administered as neoadjuvant therapy preceding radical cystectomy (RC) for muscle-invasive bladder cancer (MIBC). J Clin Oncol 2014;32(Suppl 4):324.

60. Houédé N, Pourquier P. Targeting the genetic alterations of the PI3K-AKT-mTOR pathway: its potential use in the treatment of bladder cancers. Pharmacol Ther 2015;145C:1–18.

61. Gomez-Pinillos A, Ferrari AC. mTOR signaling pathway and mTOR inhibitors in cancer therapy. Hematol Oncol Clin North Am 2012;26(3):483–505.

62. Seront E, Rottey S, Sautois B, et al. Phase II study of everolimus in patients with locally advanced or metastatic transitional cell carcinoma of the urothelial tract: clinical activity, molecular response, and biomarkers. Ann Oncol 2012;23(10):2663–70.

63. Milowsky MI, Iyer G, Regazzi AM, et al. Phase II study of everolimus in metastatic urothelial cancer. BJU Int 2013;112(4):462–70.

64. Iyer G, Hanrahan AJ, Milowsky MI, et al. Genome sequencing identifies a basis for everolimus sensitivity. Science 2012;338(6104):221.

65. Mitra AP, Lin H, Cote RJ, et al. Biomarker profiling for cancer diagnosis, prognosis and therapeutic management. Natl Med J India 2006;18(6):304–12.

66. Shariat SF, Tokunaga H, Zhou J, et al. p53, p21, pRB, and p16 expression predict clinical outcome in cystectomy with bladder cancer. J Clin Oncol 2004;22(6):1014–24.

67. Shariat SF, Lotan Y, Karakiewicz PI, et al. p53 predictive value for pT1-2 N0 disease at radical cystectomy. J Urol 2009;182(3):907–13.

68. Mitra AP, Castelao JE, Hawes D, et al. Combination of molecular alterations and smoking intensity predicts bladder cancer outcome: a report from the Los Angeles Cancer Surveillance Program. Cancer 2013;119(4):756–65.

69. Esrig D, Elmajian D, Groshen S, et al. Accumulation of nuclear p53 and tumor progression in bladder cancer. N Engl J Med 1994;331(19):1259–64.

70. Stadler WM, Lerner SP, Groshen S, et al. Phase III study of molecularly targeted adjuvant therapy in locally advanced urothelial cancer of the bladder based on p53 status. J Clin Oncol 2011;29(25): 3443–9.

71. Mitra AP, Lin H, Datar RH, et al. Molecular biology of bladder cancer: prognostic and clinical implications. Clin Genitourin Cancer 2006;5(1):67–77.

72. Mitra AP, Birkhahn M, Cote RJ. p53 and retinoblastoma pathways in bladder cancer. World J Urol 2007;25(6):563–71.

73. Shariat SF, Karakiewicz PI, Ashfaq R, et al. Multiple biomarkers improve prediction of bladder cancer recurrence and mortality in patients undergoing cystectomy. Cancer 2008;112(2):315–25.

74. Mitra AP, Hansel DE, Cote RJ. Prognostic value of cell-cycle regulation biomarkers in bladder cancer. Semin Oncol 2012;39(5):524–33.

75. Shariat SF, Chade DC, Karakiewicz PI, et al. Combination of multiple molecular markers can improve prognostication in patients with locally advanced and lymph node positive bladder cancer. J Urol 2010;183(1):68–75.

76. Mitra AP, Datar RH, Cote RJ. Molecular staging of bladder cancer. BJU Int 2005;96(1):7–12.

77. Finn RS, Crown JP, Lang I, et al. Final results of a randomized phase II study of PD 0332991, a cyclin-dependent kinase (CDK)-4/6 inhibitor, in combination with letrozole vs letrozole alone for first-line treatment of ER+/HER2- advanced breast cancer (PALOMA-1; TRIO-18). Cancer Res 2014; 74(Suppl 19):CT101.

78. Bochner BH, Cote RJ, Weidner N, et al. Angiogenesis in bladder cancer: relationship between microvessel density and tumor prognosis. J Natl Cancer Inst 1995;87(21):1603–12.

79. Birkhahn M, Mitra AP, Williams AJ, et al. Predicting recurrence and progression of noninvasive papillary bladder cancer at initial presentation based on quantitative gene expression profiles. Eur Urol 2010;57(1):12–20.

80. Mitra AP, Almal AA, George B, et al. The use of genetic programming in the analysis of quantitative gene expression profiles for identification of nodal status in bladder cancer. BMC Cancer 2006;6:159.

81. Hahn NM, Stadler WM, Zon RT, et al. Phase II trial of cisplatin, gemcitabine, and bevacizumab as first-line therapy for metastatic urothelial carcinoma: Hoosier Oncology Group GU 04-75. J Clin Oncol 2011;29(12):1525–30.

82. Siefker-Radtke AO, Kamat AM, Corn PG, et al. Neoadjuvant chemotherapy with DD-MVAC and bevacizumab in high-risk urothelial cancer: results from a phase II trial at the M. D. Anderson Cancer Center. J Clin Oncol 2012;30(Suppl 5):261.

83. Dreicer R, Li H, Stein M, et al. Phase 2 trial of sorafenib in patients with advanced urothelial cancer: a trial of the Eastern Cooperative Oncology Group. Cancer 2009;115(18):4090–5.

84. Sridhar SS, Winquist E, Eisen A, et al. A phase II trial of sorafenib in first-line metastatic urothelial cancer: a study of the PMH Phase II Consortium. Invest New Drugs 2011;29(5):1045–9.

85. Choueiri TK, Ross RW, Jacobus S, et al. Double-blind, randomized trial of docetaxel plus vandetanib versus docetaxel plus placebo in platinum-pretreated metastatic urothelial cancer. J Clin Oncol 2012;30(5):507–12.

86. Necchi A, Mariani L, Zaffaroni N, et al. Pazopanib in advanced and platinum-resistant urothelial cancer: an open-label, single group, phase 2 trial. Lancet Oncol 2012;13(8):810–6.

87. Azad AA, Zoubeidi A, Gleave ME, et al. Targeting heat shock proteins in metastatic castration-resistant prostate cancer. Nat Rev Urol 2015; 12(1):26–36.

88. Katsogiannou M, Andrieu C, Rocchi P. Heat shock protein 27 phosphorylation state is associated with cancer progression. Front Genet 2014;5:346.

89. Hayashi N, Peacock JW, Beraldi E, et al. Hsp27 silencing coordinately inhibits proliferation and promotes Fas-induced apoptosis by regulating the PEA-15 molecular switch. Cell Death Differ 2012; 19(6):990–1002.

90. Kamada M, So A, Muramaki M, et al. Hsp27 knockdown using nucleotide-based therapies inhibit tumor growth and enhance chemotherapy in human bladder cancer cells. Mol Cancer Ther 2007;6(1): 299–308.

91. Hadaschik BA, Jackson J, Fazli L, et al. Intravesically administered antisense oligonucleotides targeting heat-shock protein-27 inhibit the growth of non-muscle-invasive bladder cancer. BJU Int 2008;102(5):610–6.

92. OncoGenex announces results from the phase 2 Borealis-1™ trial of apatorsen in the treatment of metastatic bladder cancer. 2014. Available at: www.prnewswire.com. Accessed January 8, 2015.

93. Nishiyama T, Tachibana M, Horiguchi Y, et al. Immunotherapy of bladder cancer using autologous dendritic cells pulsed with human lymphocyte antigen-A24-specific MAGE-3 peptide. Clin Cancer Res 2001;7(1):23–31.

94. Marchand M, Punt CJ, Aamdal S, et al. Immunisation of metastatic cancer patients with MAGE-3 protein combined with adjuvant SBAS-2: a clinical report. Eur J Cancer 2003;39(1):70–7.

95. Leach DR, Krummel MF, Allison JP. Enhancement of antitumor immunity by CTLA-4 blockade. Science 1996;271(5256):1734–6.

96. Carthon BC, Wolchok JD, Yuan J, et al. Preoperative CTLA-4 blockade: tolerability and immune monitoring in the setting of a presurgical clinical trial. Clin Cancer Res 2010;16(10):2861–71.

97. Dong H, Strome SE, Salomao DR, et al. Tumor-associated B7-H1 promotes T-cell apoptosis: a potential mechanism of immune evasion. Nat Med 2002;8(8):793–800.

98. Brahmer JR, Tykodi SS, Chow LQ, et al. Safety and activity of anti-PD-L1 antibody in patients with advanced cancer. N Engl J Med 2012;366(26): 2455–65.

99. Powles T, Eder JP, Fine GD, et al. MPDL3280A (anti-PD-L1) treatment leads to clinical activity in metastatic bladder cancer. Nature 2014;515(7528):558–62.

100. Netto GJ, Epstein JI. Theranostic and prognostic biomarkers: genomic applications in urological malignancies. Pathology 2010;42(4):384–94.

101. Meeks JJ, Bellmunt J, Bochner BH, et al. A systematic review of neoadjuvant and adjuvant chemotherapy for muscle-invasive bladder cancer. Eur Urol 2012;62(3):523–33.

102. Advanced Bladder Cancer Meta-analysis Collaboration. Neoadjuvant chemotherapy in invasive bladder cancer: update of a systematic review and meta-analysis of individual patient data. Eur Urol 2005;48(2):202–5 [discussion: 205–6].

103. Cote RJ, Esrig D, Groshen S, et al. p53 and treatment of bladder cancer. Nature 1997;385(6612):123–5.

104. Waldman T, Lengauer C, Kinzler KW, et al. Uncoupling of S phase and mitosis induced by anticancer agents in cells lacking p21. Nature 1996; 381(6584):713–6.

105. Mitra AP, Cote RJ. Searching for novel therapeutics and targets: insights from clinical trials. Urol Oncol 2007;25(4):341–3.

106. Als AB, Dyrskjøt L, von der Maase H, et al. Emmprin and survivin predict response and survival following cisplatin-containing chemotherapy in patients with advanced bladder cancer. Clin Cancer Res 2007;13(15 Pt 1):4407–14.

107. Takata R, Katagiri T, Kanehira M, et al. Predicting response to methotrexate, vinblastine, doxorubicin, and cisplatin neoadjuvant chemotherapy for bladder cancers through genome-wide gene expression profiling. Clin Cancer Res 2005;11(7):2625–36.

108. Takata R, Katagiri T, Kanehira M, et al. Validation study of the prediction system for clinical response of M-VAC neoadjuvant chemotherapy. Cancer Sci 2007;98(1):113–7.

109. Kato Y, Zembutsu H, Takata R, et al. Predicting response of bladder cancers to gemcitabine and carboplatin neoadjuvant chemotherapy through genome-wide gene expression profiling. Exp Ther Med 2011;2(1):47–56.

110. Iwasaki K, Obara W, Kato Y, et al. Neoadjuvant gemcitabine plus carboplatin for locally advanced bladder cancer. Jpn J Clin Oncol 2013;43(2):193–9.

111. Bellmunt J, Paz-Ares L, Cuello M, et al. Gene expression of ERCC1 as a novel prognostic marker in advanced bladder cancer patients receiving cisplatin-based chemotherapy. Ann Oncol 2007; 18(3):522–8.

112. Hoffmann AC, Wild P, Leicht C, et al. *MDR1* and *ERCC1* expression predict outcome of patients with locally advanced bladder cancer receiving adjuvant chemotherapy. Neoplasia 2010;12(8): 628–36.

113. Font A, Taron M, Gago JL, et al. BRCA1 mRNA expression and outcome to neoadjuvant cisplatin-based chemotherapy in bladder cancer. Ann Oncol 2011;22(1):139–44.

114. Lee JK, Havaleshko DM, Cho H, et al. A strategy for predicting the chemosensitivity of human cancers and its application to drug discovery. Proc Natl Acad Sci U S A 2007;104(32):13086–91.

115. Williams PD, Cheon S, Havaleshko DM, et al. Concordant gene expression signatures predict clinical outcomes of cancer patients undergoing systemic therapy. Cancer Res 2009;69(21):8302–9.

116. Abrams J, Conley B, Mooney M, et al. National Cancer Institute's precision medicine initiatives for the new National Clinical Trials Network. In: American Society of Clinical Oncology educational book. Alexandria (VA): American Society of Clinical Oncology; 2014. p. 71–6.

117. Grossman HB, Natale RB, Tangen CM, et al. Neoadjuvant chemotherapy plus cystectomy compared with cystectomy alone for locally advanced bladder cancer. N Engl J Med 2003;349(9): 859–66.

118. Lerner SP. Targeted therapies for metastatic bladder cancer. J Urol 2015;193(1):8–9.

Neoadjuvant Therapy in Muscle-Invasive Bladder Cancer
A Model for Rational Accelerated Drug Development

Arjun V. Balar, MD[a],*, Matthew I. Milowsky, MD[b]

KEYWORDS

- Urothelial cancer • Bladder cancer • Predictive biomarkers • Neoadjuvant chemotherapy
- Cisplatin • The Cancer Genome Atlas • Immunotherapy

KEY POINTS

- Neoadjuvant cisplatin-based chemotherapy before radical cystectomy is the standard of care in the management of muscle-invasive bladder cancer.
- Pathologic response to neoadjuvant chemotherapy is prognostic for survival following radical cystectomy.
- The neoadjuvant setting is the context in which novel treatments should be tested in muscle-invasive bladder cancer and strengths unique to this paradigm include in vivo assessment of treatment effectiveness and the availability of ample pretreatment and posttreatment tumor tissue to perform correlative studies.
- Challenges inherent to the neoadjuvant paradigm include the potential requirement to coadminister novel therapy with standard chemotherapy, as well as potential delay of curative surgery.
- The neoadjuvant model is an ideal platform to test and better understand novel molecularly targeted therapy and immunotherapy in patients with bladder cancer.

INTRODUCTION

Despite 3 decades of clinical trials investigating novel agents and combinations, cisplatin-based chemotherapy remains the only therapy shown to improve survival in both muscle-invasive and metastatic urothelial cancer. Better-tolerated, more efficacious treatments are desperately needed.

The neoadjuvant setting has been a feasible and effective platform for the testing of novel therapies in a variety of solid tumors.[1–6] One of the earliest trials, the National Surgical Adjuvant Breast and Bowel Project B18 study, randomized women undergoing surgery for localized breast cancer to either neoadjuvant or adjuvant chemotherapy and demonstrated similar outcomes with both approaches but showed that neoadjuvant therapy permitted more breast-conserving surgery and allowed for correlation of pathologic response to clinical outcomes.[5]

Cisplatin-based chemotherapy in the neoadjuvant setting for muscle-invasive bladder cancer is

Financial Disclosures: None.
Funding Sources: None.
[a] Genitourinary Cancers Program, Perlmutter NYU Cancer Center, 160 East 34th Street, 8th Floor, New York, NY 10016, USA; [b] Genitourinary Oncology, Urologic Oncology Program, UNC Lineberger Comprehensive Cancer Center, 3rd Floor Physician's Office Building, 170 Manning Drive, Chapel Hill, NC 27599, USA
* Corresponding author.
E-mail address: arjun.balar@nyumc.org

Urol Clin N Am 42 (2015) 217–224
http://dx.doi.org/10.1016/j.ucl.2015.02.004
0094-0143/15/$ – see front matter © 2015 Elsevier Inc. All rights reserved.

considered the gold standard, supported by 3 randomized phase III clinical trials and a meta-analysis of 11 randomized trials and, therefore, may serve as a framework in which novel treatments can be tested in this disease. Strengths unique to the neoadjuvant approach include in vivo assessment of treatment effectiveness, access to pretreatment and posttreatment tumor tissue to allow for the study of molecular factors that predict for response or resistance, and more precise prognostic information to guide surveillance strategies and/or decisions related to investigational adjuvant therapy. Therefore, muscle-invasive bladder cancer is an ideal disease state to provide timely and accurate information regarding a novel treatment's efficacy, including mechanisms of response, thereby accelerating the identification of more effective and better-tolerated treatments.

THE NEOADJUVANT PARADIGM IN BLADDER CANCER: HOW DID WE GET HERE?

Despite definitive treatment strategies such as radical cystectomy and concurrent chemoradiotherapy for muscle-invasive bladder cancer, up to 50% of patients will develop metastatic bladder cancer, a devastating and incurable disease.[7] The proven efficacy of perioperative chemotherapy in breast and colon cancers, and the observed efficacy of chemotherapy in metastatic bladder cancer, ultimately led to the investigation of perioperative chemotherapy in muscle-invasive bladder cancer in an effort to eradicate micrometastatic disease and, ultimately, reduce the risk of recurrence and improve survival.

Perioperative chemotherapy, whether given before (neoadjuvant) or after (adjuvant) definitive local therapy, should achieve identical outcomes because the intent is to eliminate micrometastatic disease that may already be present at initial diagnosis. Micrometastases, relative to their macrometastatic counterparts, should be, in principle, more chemotherapy-sensitive and, furthermore, patients are more likely to tolerate chemotherapy in the perioperative setting compared with treatment at the time of systemic relapse. In the design of perioperative trials of chemotherapy in muscle-invasive bladder cancer there have been compelling arguments for both the adjuvant and neoadjuvant approaches.

Arguments in favor of neoadjuvant chemotherapy include (1) improved tolerability of chemotherapy before, rather than after surgery when postsurgical morbidity may be high; (2) the ability for in vivo assessment of chemotherapy effectiveness which has been shown to be prognostic for long-term disease-free survival; and (3), in the context of locally advanced disease, tumor downstaging and potentially more effective surgical resection. Clear limitations for neoadjuvant chemotherapy are the reliance on clinical rather than pathologic staging to determine its use and the lack of validated predictive biomarkers for response, potentially leading to overtreatment in some patients.

Up-front radical cystectomy eliminates the inherent limitations of clinical staging and allows for risk-adapted decision making whereby both pathologic and clinical factors, such as age, performance status, and medical comorbidities, can be used to determine if adjuvant chemotherapy is indicated. The adjuvant approach has clear strengths in this context; for instance, patients with high-risk features for recurrence can be selected for adjuvant treatment. However, radical cystectomy is a morbid surgery and, when combined with the comorbidities that commonly coexist in bladder cancer patients, surgery may pose significant obstacles to the administration of adjuvant chemotherapy.[8]

In practice, both adjuvant and neoadjuvant trials in muscle-invasive bladder cancer have been met with obstacles related to both accrual and planned treatment delivery. Nonetheless, perioperative therapy ultimately prevailed, definitively leading to a prolongation of survival in muscle-invasive bladder cancer with the collective data to date strongly favoring the neoadjuvant approach. Looking toward the future, the neoadjuvant treatment platform provides a framework for the development of novel therapies as we continually seek to improve outcomes for patients with both localized and advanced bladder cancer.

Adjuvant Chemotherapy

In muscle-invasive bladder cancer, radical cystectomy confers a 50% to 60% long-term survival rate for all-comers. Pathologic tumor stage is strongly linked to the risk of recurrence and, therefore, patients with more advanced disease, such as extravesical or lymph node involvement, have the highest risk for recurrence and, consequently, the poorest long-term survival estimated at 40% and 10%, respectively.[9] It stands to reason that these high-risk patients should be selected for clinical trials of adjuvant chemotherapy because they are most likely to derive benefit from additional treatment. Initial reports of adjuvant chemotherapy from prospective trials from single institutions, as well as retrospective studies, were promising, but ultimately led to randomized trials that closed early due to slow accrual and inadequate delivery of assigned therapy.[10-13] Currently, despite the widespread use of adjuvant chemotherapy, there is no high-level evidence to support its use.

Two relatively small, single-center experiences suggested a survival benefit with adjuvant chemotherapy although, in 1 study, subjects randomized to the observation arm were not offered salvage chemotherapy at the time of relapse.[10,11] However, subsequent reports have been mixed. A systematic review of 8 randomized trials demonstrated no benefit in survival, even for those with extravesical or lymph node involvement.[14] However, a retrospective analysis of a multicenter, international collaborative database demonstrated a significant improvement in survival associated with the use of adjuvant chemotherapy after radical cystectomy, particularly in subjects with high-risk features.[15]

More contemporary trials have continued to address the role for adjuvant chemotherapy however, each was closed prematurely due to poor accrual. An Italian multicenter study randomized subjects with high-grade pT2, pT3/4, or lymph node–positive bladder cancer to adjuvant gemcitabine and cisplatin (GC) versus observation and demonstrated no difference in disease-free or overall survival for the 194 enrolled of 610 planned patients.

Risk-adapted approaches have also led to mixed results. A European Organization for Research and Treatment of Cancer (EORTC) study focused on high-risk subjects with pT3/4 or lymph node–positive bladder cancer with randomization to adjuvant methotrexate, vinblastine, doxorubicin, and cisplatin (MVAC), high-dose MVAC, or GC versus deferred therapy at relapse. The EORTC study, presented at the 2014 American Society of Clinical Oncology Annual Meeting, demonstrated a significant improvement in progression-free survival (PFS) but not overall survival in the 284 enrolled of 660 planned subjects.[16] Median PFS was 2.9 years for the immediate and 0.9 years for the deferred treatment arms ($P<.0001$). Median overall survival was 6.8 years for the immediate and 4.6 years for the deferred treatment arms (hazard ratio [HR] 0.78, 95% CI 0.56–1.10, $P = .13$). A trial led by the Southwest Oncology Group (SWOG) and the University of Southern California that randomized subjects with p53 overexpression by immunohistochemistry to adjuvant MVAC chemotherapy versus observation was also terminated early after slow accrual and a high-rate of noncompliance with the study design. An analysis of the 499 subjects enrolled demonstrated neither a survival benefit with adjuvant chemotherapy nor a prognostic or predictive value to p53 testing.[17] The Spanish Oncology Group Trial 99/01, a randomized trial of adjuvant chemotherapy also focused on high-risk

subjects and ultimately did provide some evidence that adjuvant chemotherapy can perhaps improve survival. Subjects with pT3/4 or lymph node–positive bladder cancer were randomized to observation versus paclitaxel and GC for 4 cycles with a planned enrollment of 340 subjects. In 2007, this study was also closed early due to poor accrual. However, a preliminary analysis of the 142 subjects enrolled demonstrated a significant improvement in survival at 5 years (60% vs 30%, HR 0.44, $P<.0009$, median follow-up 51 months).[18]

A recently reported updated meta-analysis, including a total of 945 subjects from 9 randomized trials (5 previously analyzed in the 2005 meta-analysis), demonstrated a pooled HR of 0.77 ($P = .049$) for survival and an HR of 0.66 ($P = .014$) for disease-free survival, with the greatest benefit observed in subjects with lymph node involvement.[19] Criticisms of this meta-analysis include the inclusion of trials that were of poor quality and terminated early or not yet published, leaving the role for adjuvant chemotherapy in muscle-invasive bladder cancer undefined.

Neoadjuvant Therapy

Although the clinical evidence supporting the use of neoadjuvant chemotherapy in muscle-invasive bladder cancer is well established, this treatment approach remains relatively underused.[20,21] Data from 3 large randomized studies of neoadjuvant cisplatin-based therapy have demonstrated definitive evidence for a survival benefit. The pivotal SWOG 8710 study randomized 317 subjects with cT2-T4aN0 muscle-invasive bladder cancer to 3 cycles of neoadjuvant MVAC followed by radical cystectomy versus radical cystectomy alone. Radical cystectomy alone carried a 33% higher risk of death compared with treatment with combination therapy (HR 1.33; 95% CI 1.00–1.76).[6] The Medical Research Council of the United Kingdom and EORTC BA06 phase III trial randomized 976 subjects to cisplatin, methotrexate, and vinblastine (CMV) versus no therapy before definitive treatment (radical cystectomy or radiation) for muscle-invasive bladder cancer and was powered to detect a 10% absolute improvement in survival at 3 years. Data for the 484 subjects who underwent radical cystectomy at a median follow-up of 4 years did not demonstrate a significant difference in survival with a 3-year survival rate 55.5% for the chemotherapy arm versus 50% in the no chemotherapy arm ($P = .075$).[22] A recent long-term update, however, did demonstrate a significant reduction in the risk of death (HR 0.84, 95% CI 0.72–0.99, $P<.037$) corresponding to an increase in 10-year survival from

30% to 36% for subjects receiving neoadjuvant CMV.[23] Similar outcomes were observed in an additional randomized study of neoadjuvant MVAC, as well as a large meta-analysis of 11 randomized trials; therefore, neoadjuvant cisplatin-based chemotherapy before radical cystectomy is the standard of care in patients with muscle-invasive bladder cancer.[24,25]

Subgroup analysis from the SWOG-Intergroup 8710 study demonstrated that, although all subjects benefited from neoadjuvant chemotherapy, the benefit was greatest in subjects with clinical T3 or greater disease, again raising the question of whether certain high-risk patients benefit more. Further, the rate of complete response (pT0) to neoadjuvant chemotherapy (38% for neoadjuvant chemotherapy vs 15% for no chemotherapy; $P<.001$) strongly predicted improved long-term survival, with 85% of subjects with pT0 alive at 5 years. Post hoc analysis demonstrated a similar benefit for subjects who achieved eradication of the muscle-invasive component (<pT2) and negative surgical margins versus those who had residual muscle-invasive disease.[26] This seminal observation highlights the prognostic value of in vivo assessment of response to neoadjuvant chemotherapy and supports pathologic response as a meaningful clinical endpoint in neoadjuvant studies.[27–29]

GC, a standard regimen in metastatic disease, has not been prospectively evaluated in the neoadjuvant setting. Two recent neoadjuvant trials are evaluating GC but administered in a dose-dense fashion. The first, led by the Fox Chase Cancer Center, was closed early due to a high rate of vascular toxicity. The second is an ongoing trial led by Memorial Sloan-Kettering Cancer Center (MSKCC).[30,31] A retrospective report from a single institution demonstrated a similar rate of pT0 between MVAC and GC, suggesting that survival outcomes may be similar.[32] In practice, MVAC, CMV, and GC are all commonly used neoadjuvant regimens and serve as the backbone for ongoing trials incorporating novel agents (**Table 1**).

NEOADJUVANT MODEL FOR ACCELERATED RATIONAL DRUG DEVELOPMENT

The neoadjuvant platform in muscle-invasive bladder cancer provides unique strengths for the development of novel therapies within existing standards of care. These strengths include the availability of pretreatment and posttreatment tumor specimens without research-directed biopsies that lends to rapid assessment of treatment effectiveness and, moreover, the ability to perform molecular analyses to better understand the mechanisms that determine response or resistance. Inherent to this paradigm, however, are limitations such as the potential need to coadminister novel investigational therapy with a standard cisplatin-based chemotherapy backbone, as well as the possibility of delaying potentially curative surgery while administering investigational therapy that may be ineffective.

Table 1
Ongoing trials of neoadjuvant therapy in muscle-invasive bladder cancer

Sponsor	Eligibility	Regimen	Number of Subjects	Primary Endpoint	Trial Identifier
MSKCC	cT2-4a/N0	Dose-dense GC	46	<pT2	NCT01589094
MSKCC	cT2-4a/N0	GCa plus panitumumab	38	pT0	NCT01916109
Hoosier Cancer Research Network	cT2-4a/N0	Dasatinib	25	Feasibility	NCT00706641
University Hospitals Bristol NHS	cT2-4a/N0	Cisplatin and Cabazitaxel	30	<pT2	NCT01616875
SWOG	cT2-4a/N0	GC vs dose-dense MVAC	184	COXEN score correlation	NCT02177695
University of Michigan	cT2-4/N1-3	GCa and Abraxane[a] (ABI-007)	29	pT0	NCT00585689

Abbreviations: COXEN, Co-Expression Extrapolation; GCa, gemcitabine and carboplatin; NHS, National Health Service (United Kingdom).
[a] Nab-paclitaxel.

Pretreatment and Posttreatment Tumor Collection: Beyond a Biopsy

Acquiring tumor tissue at the time of diagnosis and at completion of standard cisplatin-based chemotherapy is standard in the management of muscle-invasive bladder cancer. Patients typically undergo a transurethral resection of bladder tumor (TURBT) at initial diagnosis and ultimately undergo a radical cystectomy with pelvic lymph node dissection, which, in addition to removal of the entire bladder, entails resection of the prostate and seminal vesicles in men and en bloc resection of the cervix, uterus, fallopian tubes, ovaries, and anterior vaginal wall in women. Unfortunately, pT0 is achieved in only 30% to 40% of cases. Therefore, most patients undergoing radical cystectomy after neoadjuvant chemotherapy will have residual disease. At radical cystectomy, any residual tumor should be completely resected, aiming for negative surgical margins and at least 10 pelvic lymph nodes, which has been associated with improved survival.[33–35] The value of access to this tumor tissue as a standard of care cannot be understated. Cancer is a complex disease characterized by intratumoral heterogeneity, which has major implications for drug development, and underscores the potential limitations of conventional on-treatment biopsies.[36–38] TURBT and radical cystectomy specimens uniquely allow for assessment of tumor architecture, morphology, presence of divergent differentiation and the surrounding tumor microenvironment, and also allow for selective analysis of the invasive component, the most clinically relevant portion of the tumor. In the context of neoadjuvant therapy, residual tumors in the radical cystectomy specimen can be compared with the pretreatment TURBT specimen to assess for treatment-resistant clones, which could have major implications for subsequent therapy at the time of relapse.[39] With the emergence of novel technologies, such as next-generation sequencing platforms, genome-wide analyses of tumors are not only more widely available but also timely and increasingly cost-effective, further strengthening the neoadjuvant setting as an important platform for the development of novel therapies.[40]

Assessment of Treatment Effectiveness: Defining the Appropriate Pathologic Endpoint

Pathologic response to neoadjuvant cisplatin-based chemotherapy at radical cystectomy is associated with improved long-term overall survival.[6,27] As such, modern trials of neoadjuvant chemotherapy have used pathologic response (either complete or partial) as the primary endpoint

for the identification of promising novel treatments.[28,29] The development of novel therapies, such as molecularly targeted agents and novel immunotherapies, may require revision of these endpoints because their mechanism of action may be unique and, therefore, not immediately measurable by pathologic response.

The recently reported comprehensive molecular analysis of muscle-invasive bladder cancer by The Cancer Genome Atlas revealed dysregulation in 3 main pathways examined by somatic mutation and copy-number alterations: cell cycle regulation, RTK/RAS/PI3K, and chromatin remodeling (histone-modifying genes and SWI/SNF nucleosome remodeling complex genes).[41] A significant proportion of these alterations are likely drivers and potentially actionable by currently available targeted therapies that are approved by the Food and Drug Administration (FDA) in other diseases, as well as novel agents currently in development.[42,43] Trials enrolling genetically preselected patients, designed to maximize the probability of benefit for those patients, will increasingly become the standard method for the evaluation of novel molecularly targeted therapies. In the design of neoadjuvant trials, the target rate of pathologic response to determine clinical benefit will need to be higher than in previous neoadjuvant trials involving unselected subjects.

Further, novel immunotherapies may require the use of entirely new endpoints to assess for clinical benefit. For instance, in a presurgical trial of ipilimumab, a cytotoxic T lymphocyte–associated antigen 4 (CTLA-4) blocking antibody FDA-approved in advanced melanoma, in muscle-invasive bladder cancer patients undergoing radical cystectomy, the surgical specimens for all 12 patients enrolled demonstrated an increase in infiltration of CD4+ICOS[hi] T cells in the tumor as well as in the peripheral circulation compared with baseline.[44] CTLA-4 is a coinhibitory receptor on CD8+ T cells and its inhibition by ipilimumab promotes antitumor T-cell priming, enhancing tumor recognition by T cells. The pathologic observations in this presurgical trial have previously been associated with improved survival in a small retrospective cohort of subjects with advanced melanoma and may be a pharmacodynamic biomarker of ipilimumab therapy.[44,45] With the recently reported promising efficacy in advanced bladder cancer of blocking antibodies targeting programmed cell death receptor (PD)-1 signaling, another coinhibitory receptor expressed on CD8+ effector T cells, revision of prior definitions of clinical benefit may be needed as these therapies make their way to localized muscle-invasive disease.[46] There is substantial excitement about the activity of anti-PD-1 and PD ligand (PD-L)1 blocking antibodies in advanced bladder cancer but there is much to be learned, including the durability of responses observed thus far. The antitumor host immune response is dynamic and complex and, therefore, there are significant challenges ahead in the identification of validated predictive biomarkers for efficacy of novel immune agents. In this context, radical cystectomy specimens after neoadjuvant immunotherapy-containing regimens provide a unique opportunity to better understand mechanisms of immune response. For instance, the quantity, location, and subtypes of tumor infiltrating lymphocytes can be characterized and compared in both TURBT and radical cystectomy specimens, which could inform the efficacy of immune-targeted therapy as well as prognosis.[47]

A variety of other immunologic correlates may be performed, including functional assays such as harvesting of lymphocytes from tumor-draining lymph nodes at the time of radical cystectomy to assess immune recognition of residual tumor and correlate to outcomes.[48] With the emergence of immune checkpoint inhibitors, as well as other novel immunotherapies such as cancer vaccines and adoptive T-cell therapies, neoadjuvant trials can also serve as hypothesis-generating endeavors, providing mechanistic insights into the immunotherapy used in that trial. The neoadjuvant platform will be vital for the development of novel therapies in bladder cancer as we move beyond cytotoxic chemotherapy.[49]

Challenges in Using the Neoadjuvant Paradigm

Cisplatin-based neoadjuvant chemotherapy as a treatment standard also poses certain limitations for the development of novel therapies in muscle-invasive bladder cancer. First, novel treatments may be coadministered with a cisplatin-containing chemotherapy backbone, which may confound both the efficacy and tolerability of a novel therapeutic. If the focus is instead turned toward cisplatin-ineligible patients, time on treatment with a novel therapeutic may be less than optimal owing to concerns related to delaying a potentially curative surgery. However, these studies, essentially serving as biomarker trials, if promising, could inform the schedule and dosing of subsequent efficacy studies with a longer treatment time. Finally, despite the level 1 evidence for the use of neoadjuvant chemotherapy in muscle-invasive bladder cancer, utilization is poor, due to both patient and clinician factors that may pose a challenge to recruitment to neoadjuvant studies.[50] Nonetheless, issues related to the

conduct of neoadjuvant studies, as well as optimal study design, will need to be addressed if the neoadjuvant platform is to be a successful method for the identification of novel therapies in bladder cancer.

SUMMARY

Technological advances leading to major breakthroughs in the understanding of the molecular landscape of cancer and the emergence of novel immunotherapies have given new hope for the identification of more effective and better-tolerated therapies for patients afflicted with this deadly disease. As biomarker-selected trials become increasingly the standard method by which new agents are tested in this modern era, novel trial designs will be required to more rapidly and efficiently identify promising treatments and the neoadjuvant setting is the ideal platform for this discovery. In muscle-invasive bladder cancer, neoadjuvant therapy as a standard of care positions it well for the development of novel therapies, although challenges inherent to this paradigm will need to be addressed if this method is to be successful. The recently opened SWOG 1314 Co-expression Extrapolation (COXEN) Program to Predict Chemotherapy Response randomized neoadjuvant trial that aims to correlate a subject's COXEN score to pathologic response rate, with an ultimate goal of identifying predictive biomarkers for benefit from neoadjuvant chemotherapy, is an important first step in using the neoadjuvant model as a means to improve outcomes for patients with bladder cancer.

REFERENCES

1. Foxtrot Collaborative Group. Feasibility of preoperative chemotherapy for locally advanced, operable colon cancer: the pilot phase of a randomised controlled trial. Lancet Oncol 2012;13:1152–60.
2. Song WA, Zhou NK, Wang W, et al. Survival benefit of neoadjuvant chemotherapy in non-small cell lung cancer: an updated meta-analysis of 13 randomized control trials. J Thorac Oncol 2010;5:510–6.
3. Robova H, Rob L, Halaska MJ, et al. High-dose density neoadjuvant chemotherapy in bulky IB cervical cancer. Gynecol Oncol 2013;128:49–53.
4. Tajima H, Ohta T, Kitagawa H, et al. Pilot study of neoadjuvant chemotherapy with gemcitabine and oral S-1 for resectable pancreatic cancer. Exp Ther Med 2012;3:787–92.
5. Fisher B, Bryant J, Wolmark N, et al. Effect of preoperative chemotherapy on the outcome of women with operable breast cancer. J Clin Oncol 1998;16:2672–85.

6. Grossman HB, Natale RB, Tangen CM, et al. Neoadjuvant chemotherapy plus cystectomy compared with cystectomy alone for locally advanced bladder cancer. N Engl J Med 2003;349:859–66.

7. Stein JP, Lieskovsky G, Cote R, et al. Radical cystectomy in the treatment of invasive bladder cancer: long-term results in 1,054 patients. J Clin Oncol 2001;19:666–75.

8. Donat SM, Shabsigh A, Savage C, et al. Potential impact of postoperative early complications on the timing of adjuvant chemotherapy in patients undergoing radical cystectomy: a high-volume tertiary cancer center experience. Eur Urol 2009;55: 177–85.

9. Sternberg CN, Donat SM, Bellmunt J, et al. Chemotherapy for bladder cancer: treatment guidelines for neoadjuvant chemotherapy, bladder preservation, adjuvant chemotherapy, and metastatic cancer. Urology 2007;69:62–79.

10. Skinner DG, Daniels JR, Russell CA, et al. The role of adjuvant chemotherapy following cystectomy for invasive bladder cancer: a prospective comparative trial. J Urol 1991;145:459–64 [discussion: 464–57].

11. Stockle M, Meyenburg W, Wellek S, et al. Advanced bladder cancer (stages pT3b, pT4a, pN1 and pN2): improved survival after radical cystectomy and 3 adjuvant cycles of chemotherapy. Results of a controlled prospective study. J Urol 1992;148:302–6 [discussion: 306–7].

12. Logothetis CJ, Johnson DE, Chong C, et al. Adjuvant cyclophosphamide, doxorubicin, and cisplatin chemotherapy for bladder cancer: an update. J Clin Oncol 1988;6:1590–6.

13. Logothetis CJ, Johnson DE, Chong C, et al. Adjuvant chemotherapy of bladder cancer: a preliminary report. J Urol 1988;139:1207–11.

14. Meeks JJ, Bellmunt J, Bochner BH, et al. A Systematic Review of Neoadjuvant and Adjuvant Chemotherapy for Muscle-invasive Bladder Cancer. Eur Urol 2012;62:523–33.

15. Svatek RS, Shariat SF, Lasky RE, et al. The effectiveness of off-protocol adjuvant chemotherapy for patients with urothelial carcinoma of the urinary bladder. Clin Cancer Res 2010;16:4461–7.

16. Sternberg CN, Kerst JM, Fossa SD, et al. Final results of EORTC intergroup randomized phase III trial comparing immediate versus deferred chemotherapy after radical cystectomy in patients with pT3T4 and/or N+ M0 transitional cell carcinoma (TCC) of the bladder. American Society of Clinical Oncology Annual Meeting. J Clin Oncol 2014; 32(Suppl):5s [abstr 4500].

17. Stadler WM, Lerner SP, Groshen S, et al. Phase III study of molecularly targeted adjuvant therapy in locally advanced urothelial cancer of the bladder based on p53 status. J Clin Oncol 2011;29:3443–9.

18. Paz-Ares LG, Solsona E, Esteban E, et al. Randomized phase III trial comparing adjuvant paclitaxel/gemcitabine/cisplatin (PGC) to observation in patients with resected invasive bladder cancer: results of the Spanish oncology genitourinary group (SOGUG) 99/01 study. J Clin Oncol 2010; 28(Suppl):18s [abstr LBA4518].

19. Leow JJ, Martin-Doyle W, Rajagopal PS, et al. Adjuvant chemotherapy for invasive bladder cancer: a 2013 updated systematic review and meta-analysis of randomized trials. Eur Urol 2014;66:42–54.

20. Burger M, Mulders P, Witjes W. Use of neoadjuvant chemotherapy for muscle-invasive bladder cancer is low among major European centres: results of a feasibility questionnaire. Eur Urol 2012; 61:1070–1.

21. Raj GV, Karavadia S, Schlomer B, et al. Contemporary use of perioperative cisplatin-based chemotherapy in patients with muscle-invasive bladder cancer. Cancer 2011;117:276–82.

22. Advanced Bladder Cancer (ABC) Meta-analysis Collaboration. Adjuvant chemotherapy in invasive bladder cancer: a systematic review and meta-analysis of individual patient data Advanced Bladder Cancer (ABC) Meta-analysis Collaboration. Eur Urol 2005;48:189–99 [discussion: 199–201].

23. Griffiths G, Hall R, Sylvester R, et al. International phase III trial assessing neoadjuvant cisplatin, methotrexate, and vinblastine chemotherapy for muscle-invasive bladder cancer: long-term results of the BA06 30894 trial. J Clin Oncol 2011;29:2171–7.

24. Advanced Bladder Cancer (ABC) Meta-analysis Collaboration. Neoadjuvant chemotherapy in invasive bladder cancer: a systematic review and meta-analysis. Lancet 2003;361:1927–34.

25. Kitamura H, Tsukamoto T, Masumori N, et al. Randomized phase III trial of neoadjuvant chemotherapy (NAC) with methotrexate, doxorubicin, vinblastine, and cisplatin (MVAC) followed by radical cystectomy (RC) compared with RC alone for invasive bladder cancer (BC): Japan Clinical Oncology Group Study, JCOG0209. J Clin Oncol 2013; 31(Suppl 6) [abstract: 249].

26. Sonpavde G, Goldman BH, Speights VO, et al. Quality of pathologic response and surgery correlate with survival for patients with completely resected bladder cancer after neoadjuvant chemotherapy. Cancer 2009;115:4104–9.

27. Splinter TA, Pavone-Macaluso M, Jacqmin D, et al. A European Organization for Research and Treatment of Cancer—Genitourinary Group phase 2 study of chemotherapy in stage T3-4N0-XM0 transitional cell cancer of the bladder: evaluation of clinical response. J Urol 1992;148:1793–6.

28. Plimack ER, Hoffman-Censits JH, Viterbo R, et al. Accelerated methotrexate, vinblastine, doxorubicin, and cisplatin is safe, effective, and efficient

neoadjuvant treatment for muscle-invasive bladder cancer: results of a multicenter phase II study with molecular correlates of response and toxicity. J Clin Oncol 2014;32:1895–901.

29. Choueiri TK, Jacobus S, Bellmunt J, et al. Neoadjuvant dose-dense methotrexate, vinblastine, doxorubicin, and cisplatin with pegfilgrastim support in muscle-invasive urothelial cancer: pathologic, radiologic, and biomarker correlates. J Clin Oncol 2014; 32:1889–94.

30. Neoadjuvant dose dense gemcitabine and cisplatin (dd gc) in patients with muscle-invasive bladder cancer. Available at: http://clinicaltrials.gov/ct2/show/NCT01589094?term=dose+dense+gemcitabine+and+cisplatin&rank=1. Accessed August 20, 2012.

31. Plimack E, Hoffman-Censits J, Kutikov A, et al. Neoadjuvant dose-dense gemcitabine and cisplatin (DDGC) in patients (pts) with muscle-invasive bladder cancer (MIBC): final results of a multicenter phase II study. Chicago (IL): ASCO Annual Meeting. May 29-June 3 2014.

32. Skeldon SC, Semotiuk K, Aronson M, et al. Patients with Lynch syndrome mismatch repair gene mutations are at higher risk for not only upper tract urothelial cancer but also bladder cancer. Eur Urol 2013;63:379–85.

33. Herr HW, Faulkner JR, Grossman HB, et al. Surgical factors influence bladder cancer outcomes: a cooperative group report. J Clin Oncol 2004;22:2781–9.

34. Leissner J, Hohenfellner R, Thuroff JW, et al. Lymphadenectomy in patients with transitional cell carcinoma of the urinary bladder; significance for staging and prognosis. BJU Int 2000;85:817–23.

35. Koppie TM, Serio AM, Vickers AJ, et al. Age-adjusted Charlson comorbidity score is associated with treatment decisions and clinical outcomes for patients undergoing radical cystectomy for bladder cancer. Cancer 2008;112:2384–92.

36. Xu X, Hou Y, Yin X, et al. Single-cell exome sequencing reveals single-nucleotide mutation characteristics of a kidney tumor. Cell 2012;148:886–95.

37. Gerlinger M, Rowan AJ, Horswell S, et al. Intratumor heterogeneity and branched evolution revealed by multiregion sequencing. N Engl J Med 2012;366: 883–92.

38. Bajorin DF, Dodd PM, Mazumdar M, et al. Long-term survival in metastatic transitional-cell carcinoma and prognostic factors predicting outcome of therapy. J Clin Oncol 1999;17:3173–81.

39. Bellmunt J, Pons F, Orsola A. Molecular determinants of response to cisplatin-based neoadjuvant chemotherapy. Curr Opin Urol 2013;23:466–71.

40. Tripathy D, Harnden K, Blackwell K, et al. Next generation sequencing and tumor mutation profiling: are we ready for routine use in the oncology clinic? BMC Med 2014;12:140.

41. The Cancer Genome Atlas Research Network. Comprehensive molecular characterization of urothelial bladder carcinoma. Nature 2014;507: 315–22.

42. Iyer G, Al-Ahmadie H, Schultz N, et al. Prevalence and co-occurrence of actionable genomic alterations in high-grade bladder cancer. J Clin Oncol 2013;31:3133–40.

43. Iyer G, Hanrahan AJ, Milowsky MI, et al. Genome sequencing identifies a basis for everolimus sensitivity. Science 2012;338:221.

44. Carthon BC, Wolchok JD, Yuan J, et al. Preoperative CTLA-4 blockade: tolerability and immune monitoring in the setting of a presurgical clinical trial. Clin Cancer Res 2010;16:2861–71.

45. Ng Tang D, Shen Y, Sun J, et al. Increased frequency of ICOS+ CD4 T cells as a pharmacodynamic biomarker for anti-CTLA-4 therapy. Cancer Immunol Res 2013;1:229–34.

46. Powles T, Eder JP, Fine GD, et al. MPDL3280A (anti-PD-L1) treatment leads to clinical activity in metastatic bladder cancer. Nature 2014;515:558–62.

47. Galon J, Costes A, Sanchez-Cabo F, et al. Type, density, and location of immune cells within human colorectal tumors predict clinical outcome. Science 2006;313:1960–4.

48. Clay TM, Hobeika AC, Mosca PJ, et al. Assays for monitoring cellular immune responses to active immunotherapy of cancer. Clin Cancer Res 2001;7: 1127–35.

49. Horig H, Pullman W. From bench to clinic and back: Perspective on the 1st IQPC translational research conference. J Transl Med 2004;2:44.

50. Cowan NG, Chen Y, Downs TM, et al. Neoadjuvant chemotherapy use in bladder cancer: a survey of current practice and opinions. Adv Urol 2014;2014: 746298.

Novel Biomarkers to Predict Response and Prognosis in Localized Bladder Cancer

Ilaria Lucca, MD[a,b], Michela de Martino, PhD[a],
Tobias Klatte, MD[a], Shahrokh F. Shariat, MD[a,c,d],*

KEYWORDS

- Nonmuscle invasive bladder cancer • Diagnostic biomarkers • Prognostic biomarkers • DNA
- RNA • Protein • Urine

KEY POINTS

- Urothelial carcinoma of the bladder (UCB) is the most expensive solid tumor to treat because of its high recurrence rate and the need of continued cystoscopic surveillance.
- Cystoscopy has a high sensitivity and specificity, but is a costly and invasive procedure; urinary cytology is noninvasive and highly specific and shows very low overall sensitivity, in particular in low-grade nonmuscle invasive bladder cancer (NMIBC).
- Several biomarkers may have better sensitivity than voided urinary cytology, but they are not accurate enough to replace cystoscopy and cytology.
- *NMP22, BTA*, ImmunoCyt/uCyt+ and UroVysion/FISH have been approved by the Food and Drug Administration for screening and follow-up of patients with NMIBC in combination with cystoscopy.
- The long interval required for validation, testing, and approval of the assays and the lack of standardization could explain the present failure of biomarkers to predict NMIBC development, recurrence, and progression.

INTRODUCTION

Urothelial carcinoma of the bladder (UCB) is the most expensive solid tumor to treat because of its high recurrence rate and need of continued surveillance, with an estimated annual cost of $3.7 billion in the United States.[1] More than 400,000 patients are newly diagnosed with UCB worldwide every year, and more than 150,000 die from the disease.[2]

The standard evaluation of a suspected UCB consists of cystoscopy and urinary cytology.[3] Although cystoscopy has a high sensitivity and

Funding Sources: Development fund of the CHUV-University Hospital, European Urological Scholarship Programme (I. Lucca); Oesterreichische Nationalbank Anniversary Fund (project number: 15363/2013), Medical-Scientific Fund of the Mayor of the City of Vienna (project number: 14069/2014) (T. Klatte); Nil (M. de Martino, S. Shariat).
Conflict of Interest: Nil.
[a] Department of Urology, Comprehensive Cancer Center, Vienna General Hospital, Medical University of Vienna, Währinger Gürtel 18-20, Vienna A-1090, Austria; [b] Department of Urology, Centre Hospitalier Universitaire Vaudois, Rue du Bugnon 46, Lausanne CH-1010, Switzerland; [c] Department of Urology, University of Texas Southwestern Medical Center, 1801 Inwood Road, Dallas, TX 75235, USA; [d] Department of Urology, Weill Cornell Medical College, New York-Presbyterian Hospital, Cornell University, 1300 York Avenue, New York, NY 10065, USA
* Corresponding author. Department of Urology, Comprehensive Cancer Center, Vienna General Hospital, Medical University Vienna, Währinger Gürtel 18-20, Vienna A-1090, Austria.
E-mail address: sfshariat@gmail.com

Urol Clin N Am 42 (2015) 225–233
http://dx.doi.org/10.1016/j.ucl.2015.01.004
0094-0143/15/$ – see front matter © 2015 Elsevier Inc. All rights reserved.

urologic.theclinics.com

specificity, it is a costly and invasive procedure, with a risk of complications, such as urinary infections, pain, and bleeding. Urinary cytology has a low overall sensitivity rate of only 33% to 48%, but a higher specificity of 86% to 90% in the detection of nonmuscle invasive bladder cancer (NMIBC).[4,5] Its predictive accuracy improves in high-grade tumors to approximately 90%, whereas it does not go beyond 60% in low-grade NMIBC.[6] Urinary cytology after bladder washing seems to have a higher sensitivity than from voided urine.[7]

In UCB, the TNM staging together with various prognostic models, such as the European Organization for the Research and Treatment of Cancer (EORTC) and Spanish Urological Club for Oncological Treatment (CUETO) scoring systems, allow defining the risk of recurrence and progression after the surgery.[3,8] However, among patients with UCB staged similarly, there is still a considerable variation in rates of recurrence, disease progression, and response to treatment. Therefore, biomarkers are needed to improve prognostication.

Intense work is being done in the field of NMIBC biomarkers with the main goals of reducing the number of invasive cystoscopic evaluations through early diagnosis and identifying those patients with a higher risk of disease progression. The identification of valuable NMIBC biomarkers would improve our understanding of the biological pathways involved in the genesis and progression of the tumor, but would also add information about UCB outcomes.

A biomarker is an indicator of biological and pathogenic processes or pharmaceutical responses to a therapeutic intervention.[9] The ideal biomarker should be noninvasive, rapid to analyze, objective, easy to perform, sensitive, specific, reproducible, and, above all, cost-effective. However, to date, the available biomarkers are all lacking one or more of these characteristics. Several biomarkers showed a higher sensitivity than voided urinary cytology, but they are not accurate enough to replace it. Indeed, although several studies have been published on NMIBC biomarkers in recent years, none of them is recommended for use in clinical practice.

The classification of UCB biomarkers is relatively complex. They could be classified according to (1) the sample used for their identification, (2) their objective, (3) the biomolecule, or (4) the type of measurements applied (**Fig. 1**).[10]

Because the literature on this topic is vast, the aim of this review was to provide a summary of the most relevant biomarkers investigated in the last period as predictor of NMIBC, recurrence, and aggressiveness.

DIAGNOSTIC BIOMARKERS FOR EARLY DETECTION OF NONMUSCLE INVASIVE BLADDER CANCER

Diagnostic biomarkers aim to detect the disease in symptomatic patients or in those having an increased risk, if possible at early stages.[11] NMIBC is an attractive tumor for screening because of its well-known risk factors and its favorable outcomes when diagnosed at early stages. Macrohematuria is the most common symptom, but it is not specific and is not related to the pathologic stage. Madeb and Messing[12] screened 1575 men aged 50 years or older without a history of UCB,

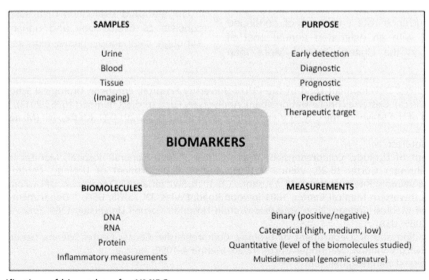

Fig. 1. Classification of biomarkers for NMIBC.

hematuria, or previous treatment with pelvic radiation therapy for hematuria. Although 6% to 10% of men with hematuria were diagnosed with UCB, hemoglobin dipsticks had a positive predictive value of only 8.1%. It has been hypothesized that a combination of home hematuria urinary testing and a panel of biomarkers may improve the sensitivity and specificity of the screening. The Bladder Cancer Urine Marker Project (BLU-P) tested a total of 1747 Dutch men with a home hematuria test followed by a molecular marker panel, which included nuclear matrix protein 22 (NMP22), microsatellite analysis (MA), the fibroblast growth factor receptor 3 (FGFR3) mutation snapshot assay, and a custom methylation-specific (MLPA) test.[13] The specificity and sensitivity of any positive molecular test were 95.9% and 80.0%, respectively. However, of the 71 men who finally underwent cystoscopy, only 4 UCBs and 1 upper tract urothelial carcinoma were detected, showing a lack of benefit of this combined screening approach in a large unselected asymptomatic population.

Protein Biomarkers

Several studies have reported the association of urinary protein biomarkers and UCB, leading to the Food and Drug Administration (FDA) approval of NMP22, bladder tumor antigen (BTA), and ImmunoCyt/uCyt+ for screening and follow-up in combination with cystoscopy.

NMP22 is a protein found in the nuclear matrix and is involved in replication and gene expression. The sensitivity and specificity of the urinary NMP22 test to detect UCB is approximately 68% and 79%, respectively.[14–16] The test is commercially available and detects urinary levels of the nuclear mitotic apparatus protein, which is elevated in the urine of patients with UCB. However, a high rate of false-positive tests has been reported, often due to macrohematuria, urinary tract infections, and instrumentation. Ponsky and colleagues[17] showed that benign inflammatory or infectious conditions, renal or bladder calculi, current or recent history of foreign body in the urinary tract, any bowel interposition segment, and other genitourinary cancers are responsible for reducing the positive predictive value and the specificity. Based on an experimental model, Miyake and colleagues[18] suggested that urinary NMP22 assays may diagnose UCB by counting the amount of cell turnover as consequences of surface shedding from bladder tumors rather than identifying a specific tumor antigen. That would explain the false-negative NMP22 tests in those with reduced urinary cellularity due to the characteristic of the tumor or an error in sampling. Moreover, concentrated urine may be also responsible for false-positive tests because of an overestimation of NMP22 levels.[19] Taken together, NMP22 cannot be considered an alternative to cystoscopy.

The BTA test detects the human complement factor H-related protein, which seems to prevent cell lysis in UCB.[20] The original BTA test (Bard Diagnostics, Redmond, WA) was taken off the market because of its very low specificity and sensitivity.[21] Two tests are currently available, the BTA stat and BTA TRAK (Polymedco, Cortlandt Manor, NY). Although the first is qualitative and gives an immediate result, the second is quantitative and requires experienced laboratory processing. The overall BTA sensitivity is higher than urinary cytology (61%–67%), but the specificity seems to be lower (75%–78%).[4,22] The presence of blood in the urine interferes with the BTA tests, causing a high rate of false-positive results due to the cross-reactivity to antigens on red blood cells.[23] Some investigators have suggested the use of BTA as serum biomarker, measuring complement factor H introduced by bleeding.[24]

ImmunoCyt/uCyt+ (Scimedx, Denville, NJ) is approved by the FDA for the follow-up of patients with NMIBC. It combines 3 monoclonal antibodies and operates as a second-level test in case of atypical urinary cytology. Odisho and colleagues[25] performed ImmunoCyt/uCyt+ tests on 506 voided urine samples with atypical urinary cytology. For low-grade UCB, the sensitivity, specificity, and negative predictive value were 75%, 50%, and 82%, respectively. For high-grade UCB, the values were comparable (74%, 44%, and 79%, respectively). Moreover, Têtu and colleagues[26] showed a significant improvement of the urinary cytology sensitivity when combined with ImmunoCyt/uCyt+, with a sensitivity of 78% in Ta, 83% in T1, and 100% in carcinoma in situ.

Chromosome Biomarkers

Another FDA-approved urinary biomarker is UroVysion (Abbott Laboratories, Abbott Park, IL), a multitarget fluorescence in situ hybridization (FISH) assay that detects aneuploidy in chromosomes 3, 7, and 17 as well as focal loss of 9p21 containing the p16 tumor-suppressor gene.[27] A meta-analysis of 14 studies involving 2477 UroVysion-FISH tests found an overall sensitivity of 86% (82%–89%) for UroVysion compared with 61% (56%–66%) for urinary cytology.[28] However, positive FISH did not reach the level of evidence for the initial diagnosis of UCB. In patients with NMIBC with positive cytology but negative cystoscopy, the prediction of disease occurrence or recurrence is challenging. In a study investigating 243 patients with NMIBC with atypical urinary cytology, a positive UroVysion-FISH test was a significant predictor of recurrence (hazard ratio 2.35, $P = .001$) in multivariate analysis.[29] Finally, Seideman and colleagues[30] showed that patients with NMIBC with atypical urinary cytology and positive UroVysion-FISH had a shorter time to recurrence compared with those with a negative UroVysion-FISH (12.6 vs 17.9 months), even when cystoscopy was negative.

DNA Methylation Biomarkers

DNA methylation is one of the most studied epigenetic mechanisms, which commonly occurs in CpG-rich regions that are located in the promoter regions and lead to gene inactivation.[31] Because CpG hypermethylation does not occur in normal cells, many methylated genes have been linked to UCB pathways.[32–38] The detection of methylation biomarkers has several advantages over conventional genetic markers because of their high degree of specificity, which is important when DNA is available in limited quantities (eg, from biological fluids such as urine). Moreover, they play a role in both diagnosis and prognosis of UCB. Su and colleagues[39] built a panel of biomarkers, including a combination of a transcription factor (SOX1), a specific LINE-1 element, and interleukin-1 receptor-associated kinase 3 (IRAK3), which could detect a higher rate of early recurrences than urinary cytology and cystoscopy. DNA methylated biomarkers, such as OTX1, ONECUT2, and OSR1, have been studied in combination with FGFR3 assays, showing a sensitivity of 79% and a specificity of 77% in patients with NMIBC.[40]

Because DNA methylation is involved in UCB pathogenesis, numerous promoters of DNA hypermethylation are being investigated (ie, tumor-suppressor genes, proto-oncogenes, genes involved in cell adhesion, and genes regulating the cell cycle).[41,42] In a recent study, histone deacetylases (HDAC)-1 and HDAC-2 overexpression was associated with the development of high-grade NMIBC, suggesting a potential role of HDAC inhibitors as chemotherapeutics.[43] Moreover, downregulated KLF4 has been found to promote DNA hypermethylation and may be associated with a higher risk of early recurrence and disease progression.[44]

Micro RNA Biomarkers

Micro RNAs (miRNAs) are short noncoding RNA molecules of 18 to 22 nucleotides that are able to modulate posttranscriptional protein expression. Upregulation or downregulation of miRNAs may influence UCB tumorigenesis by acting as oncogenes or tumor-suppressor genes. A total of 2216 miRNAs have been registered so far.[45] Most miRNA studies focus on tissue samples, whereas only one-third is on urine samples. Low-grade UCB is characterized by miRNA downregulation, whereas in high-grade UCB, there is typically miRNA upregulation.[46] A recent meta-analysis identified 15 miRNAs as the most promising diagnostic and prognostic UCB biomarkers, of which 11 were upregulated (miRNA-96, miRNA-138, miRNA-126, miRNA-182, miRNA-143, miRNA-222, miRNA-21, miRNA-133b, miRNA-518c-5p, miRNA-452, and miRNA-129) and 4 were downregulated (miRNA-200c, miRNA-99a, miRNA-100, and miRNA-29c).[47] Among them, miRNA-99a expression was inversely correlated with the aggressiveness of UCB, suggesting a role of miRNA-99a as tumor suppressor.[48] Also miRNA-100 might act as a tumor suppressor. Indeed, when artificially reintroduced in tumor tissue, it is able to suppress cell proliferation and motility, inducing cell-cycle arrest in vitro.[49] Finally, some promising miRNAs, such as miRNA-141 and miRNA-639, have been recently studied in plasma, but final results showed no differences in serum levels between patients with UCB and controls.[50]

Messenger RNA Biomarkers

Survivin, also known as BIRC5 or EPR-1, has a pivotal role in promoting cell proliferation and preventing apoptosis. Its sensitivity and specificity to predict UCB have been estimated at approximately 76% to 78% and 82% to 95%, respectively, and when survivin tests are combined with urinary cytology, the accuracy increases significantly.[51–53] Moreover, patients with NMIBC expressing high survivin levels have shown a lower risk of disease recurrence.[54] Another interesting mRNA biomarker is Aurora A kinase (AURKA), a cell-cycle–associated serine/threonine kinase involved in genetic stability. The AURKA overexpression seems to be specific of UCB tissue and in voided urine samples may be associated with higher UCB stage and grade, and worse survival.[6]

PROGNOSTIC BIOMARKERS IN NONMUSCLE INVASIVE BLADDER CANCER

In NMIBC, presence of carcinoma in situ, tumor stage and grade, tumor size, and numbers of lesions are established variables to predict disease recurrence and progression. It has been estimated that 10% to 20% of patients progress to a muscle-invasive stage.[55,56] New prognostic biomarkers that identify patients with a high risk of progression, and may therefore be candidates for a more aggressive therapy, are needed.

Inflammatory Biomarkers

Inflammation plays a pivotal role in the development and progression of UCB.[57,58] It is commonly accepted that the tumor microenvironment triggers the release of cytokines, subsequently influencing the systemic inflammatory response.[59] Measurements of systemic inflammatory response represent valuable, reproducible, and inexpensive prognostic biomarkers. According to a recent meta-analysis, inflammatory cells, UCB-costimulatory molecules, serum cytokines, and the C-reactive protein were all significantly associated with survival.[60]

Some inflammatory measurements have been combined in ratios to improve their prognostic value. A high neutrophil-to-lymphocyte ratio (NLR) has been associated with poor survival and higher risk of disease recurrence in NMIBC. Mano and colleagues[61] estimated a 3-year progression-free survival rate of 61% in patients with NMIBC with a preoperative NLR greater than 2.41, compared with a rate of 84% in patients with an NLR of 2.41 or less ($P = .004$).

Cell Cycle and Adhesion Markers

In the past decade, several molecular biomarkers have been identified as potential predictors of UCB progression to an invasive stage.[62] The p53 protein is a well-known tumor-suppressor protein with a crucial role in the prevention of genomic mutations. Besides its role in predicting early recurrence, several studies showed an association between p53 overexpression and UCB progression.[63,64] Shariat and colleagues[65] studied p53 in combination with other molecular markers (pRB, p21, and p27). The investigators found that a high number of altered biomarkers was significantly associated with an increased risk of disease recurrence ($P = .011$) and progression ($P = .005$).

Deletions of the long arm of chromosome 9 and mutations in FGFR3, H-RAS, and PI3K also may influence the development of UCB.[66] Lindgren and colleagues[67] found higher frequency of FGFR3 mutations in low-grade NMIBC (80%) than in high-grade NMIBC (less than 10%), suggesting a protection role of FGFR3 against disease progression. On the other hand, others failed to show that deletions of the long arm of chromosome 9 and mutations of HRAS are associated with disease progression.[68,69]

CD44v6 is a promising protein involved in cell migration and adhesion. It has been shown that CD44v6 expression is lower in high-grade compared with low-grade lesions, and is associated with an increased risk of disease recurrence.[70] CD44v6 seems to specifically target UCB, as no correlation with other bladder tumor histologies, tumor size, and patient characteristics were observed.[71]

Hypoxia-Related and Angiogenesis-Related Biomarkers

Several studies have shown an association of worse outcomes with altered angiogenesis-related markers. Shariat and colleagues[72] showed that the overexpression of vascular endothelial growth factor (VEGF) and basic fibroblast growth factor, as well as the decreased expression of thrombospondin 1 were associated with higher UCB stages, lymphovascular invasion, and lymph node metastasis. Alterations of VEGF are influenced by the expression of its 2 receptors, VEGF-receptor-1 (VEGFR1) and 2 (VEGFR2). Although VEGFR2 seems to be overexpressed in muscle-invasive bladder cancer, VEGFR1 tends to be overexpressed in NMIBC.[73] Finally, a recent meta-analysis of 11 studies supports the hypothesis that overexpression of VEGF in NMIBC is associated with poor prognosis.[74] CD34 is a transmembrane cell surface glycoprotein involved in tumor angiogenesis.[75] In patients with NMIBC, CD34 microvessel density has been found to be associated with recurrence after Bacillus Calmette-Guerin.[76] Another novel prognostic marker involved in angiogenesis is hyaluronoglucosaminidase 1 (HYAL-1). Based on tissue microarrays from a cohort of 178 UCB specimens, Kramer and colleagues[77] showed a significant association between HYAL-1 and disease progression to invasive stages.

Hypoxia is a stress signal during tumor growth and regulates gene expression. The carbonic anhydrase IX (CAIX) is a hypoxia-related biomarker, responsible of intracellular pH regulation and hydrogen ion (H+) flux.[78] Among NMIBC, higher CAIX expression was found to be associated with lower recurrence-free survival and a 6.5-fold higher risk of disease progression.[79] The 6-phosphofructo-2-kinase/fructose-2,6-biphosphatase 4 (PFKFB4) is also induced by hypoxia. Yun and colleagues[80] found that overexpression of PFKFB4 was significantly associated with high-stage UCB and multiple tumors compared with low stage and single tumors ($P<.05$), suggesting PFKFB4 as a new valid prognostic marker of NMIBC progression.

Finally, the ABO blood type also might influence UCB progression. One group recently showed that patients with blood type O had a higher rate of progression than those with A ($P = .031$) or B ($P = .075$).[81]

THE FUTURE OF BIOMARKERS IN THE MANAGEMENT OF NONMUSCLE INVASIVE BLADDER CANCER

Despite numerous studies on biomarkers in UCB, only a few of them have been accepted for clinical practice together with cystoscopy and urinary cytology. Several biomarkers have shown a higher sensitivity compared with urinary cytology, but they are still not accurate enough to be included in guidelines.[82] Today, there is no biomarker available that could replace cystoscopy and urinary cytology in the management of NMIBC. Yossepowitch and colleagues[83] interviewed 200 patients with a history of UCB about the expected accuracy for a biomarker. Three-quarters of the patients would accept being tested with a urinary marker alone if its sensitivity would be greater than 95%.

The long interval required for validation, testing, and approval of the assays and the lack of standardization for the development of new biomarkers could explain this failure.[84] Most known biomarkers are not reproducible, leading to contrasting biomedical and statistical results between different institutions.[85] Moreover, several studies on UCB biomarkers are limited by the statistical tests applied, their study design, the investigated cohort, the definition of end points, and laboratory methods.[86] Finally, the selection of a specific high-risk population is crucial to improve the sensitivity and specificity of biomarkers. To enhance the detection and evaluation of UCB biomarkers, Shariat and colleagues[10] proposed a 6-phase approach, composed of preclinical testing, assay development, feasibility and clinical prevalence, validation and standardization for clinical utility, independent confirmation studies, and finally impact assessment. Indeed, with this method, only a very few biomarkers would be finally approved for routine clinical practice, in the same way as pharmaceutical drugs.

Although the discovery of new biomarkers remains crucial, the creation of a panel of biomarkers ready to be tested in a large population should be the future main focus.[5,87–89] Most NMIBC biomarkers seem to be independently associated with outcomes of specific subgroups of individuals, according to their age, gender, ethnicity, and risk factors.[90–94] Therefore, the development of a panel of biomarkers seems a concrete possibility to improve the overall sensitivity and specificity as well as to predict outcomes. Mengual and colleagues[95] developed a multimarker diagnostic and prognostic urine test composed of 12+2 gene expression signature for UCB with an overall sensitivity of 98% and 79% and a specificity of 99% and 92% in discriminating between UCB

and control samples and in predicting tumor aggressiveness, respectively. Similarly, García-Baquero and colleagues[96] evaluated the DNA methylation of 18 tumor-suppressor genes in urine samples of patients with UCB, finding that CCND2, SCGB3A1, BNIP3, ID4, and RUNX3 were the most frequently methylated tumor-suppressor genes in each urine set.

REFERENCES

1. Sievert KD, Amend B, Nagele U, et al. Economic aspects of bladder cancer: what are the benefits and costs? World J Urol 2009;27(3):295–300.
2. Ferlay J, Soerjomataram I, Dikshit R, et al. Cancer incidence and mortality worldwide: sources, methods and major patterns in GLOBOCAN 2012. Int J Cancer 2015;136:E359–86.
3. Babjuk M, Burger M, Zigeuner R, et al. EAU guidelines on non-muscle-invasive urothelial carcinoma of the bladder: update 2013. Eur Urol 2013;64(4):639–53.
4. Yafi FA, Brimo F, Steinberg J, et al. Prospective analysis of sensitivity and specificity of urinary cytology and other urinary biomarkers for bladder cancer. Urol Oncol 2014. http://dx.doi.org/10.1016/j.urolonc.2014.06.008.
5. Rosser CJ, Chang M, Dai Y, et al. Urinary protein biomarker panel for the detection of recurrent bladder cancer. Cancer Epidemiol Biomarkers Prev 2014;23(7):1340–5.
6. De Martino M, Shariat SF, Hofbauer SL, et al. Aurora A Kinase as a diagnostic urinary marker for urothelial bladder cancer. World J Urol 2015;33:105–10.
7. Bolenz C, West AM, Ortiz N, et al. Urinary cytology for the detection of urothelial carcinoma of the bladder–a flawed adjunct to cystoscopy? Urol Oncol 2013;31(3):366–71.
8. Vedder MM, Márquez M, de Bekker-Grob EW, et al. Risk prediction scores for recurrence and progression of non-muscle invasive bladder cancer: an international validation in primary tumours. PLoS One 2014;9(6):e96849.
9. Biomarkers Definitions Working Group. Biomarkers and surrogate endpoints: preferred definitions and conceptual framework. Clin Pharmacol Ther 2001;69(3):89–95.
10. Shariat SF, Lotan Y, Vickers A, et al. Statistical consideration for clinical biomarker research in bladder cancer. Urol Oncol 2010;28(4):389–400.
11. Barrow TM, Michels KB. Epigenetic epidemiology of cancer. Biochem Biophys Res Commun 2014;455(1–2):70–83.
12. Madeb R, Messing EM. Long-term outcome of home dipstick testing for hematuria. World J Urol 2008;26(1):19–24.

13. Bangma CH, Loeb S, Busstra M, et al. Outcomes of a bladder cancer screening program using home hematuria testing and molecular markers. Eur Urol 2013;64(1):41–7.

14. Shariat SF, Casella R, Wians FH, et al. Risk stratification for bladder tumor recurrence, stage and grade by urinary nuclear matrix protein 22 and cytology. Eur Urol 2004;45(3):304–13 [author reply: 313].

15. Shariat SF, Casella R, Khoddami SM, et al. Urine detection of survivin is a sensitive marker for the noninvasive diagnosis of bladder cancer. J Urol 2004;171(2 Pt 1):626–30.

16. Campbell MK, Skea ZC, Sutherland AG, et al. Effectiveness and cost-effectiveness of arthroscopic lavage in the treatment of osteoarthritis of the knee: a mixed methods study of the feasibility of conducting a surgical placebo-controlled trial (the KORAL study). Health Technol Assess 2010;14(5): 1–180.

17. Ponsky LE, Sharma S, Pandrangi L, et al. Screening and monitoring for bladder cancer: refining the use of NMP22. J Urol 2001;166(1):75–8.

18. Miyake M, Goodison S, Giacoia EG, et al. Influencing factors on the NMP-22 urine assay: an experimental model. BMC Urol 2012;12:23.

19. Joung JY, Park S, Yoon H, et al. Overestimation of nuclear matrix protein 22 in concentrated urine. Urology 2013;82(5):1059–64.

20. Babjuk M, Kostírová M, Mudra K, et al. Qualitative and quantitative detection of urinary human complement factor H-related protein (BTA stat and BTA TRAK) and fragments of cytokeratins 8, 18 (UBC rapid and UBC IRMA) as markers for transitional cell carcinoma of the bladder. Eur Urol 2002;41(1):34–9.

21. Johnston B, Morales A, Emerson L, et al. Rapid detection of bladder cancer: a comparative study of point of care tests. J Urol 1997;158(6):2098–101.

22. Guo A, Wang X, Gao L, et al. Bladder tumour antigen (BTA stat) test compared to the urine cytology in the diagnosis of bladder cancer: a meta-analysis. Can Urol Assoc J 2014;8(5–6):E347–52.

23. Lüdecke G, Pilatz A, Hauptmann A, et al. Comparative analysis of sensitivity to blood in the urine for urine-based point-of-care assays (UBC rapid, NMP22 BladderChek and BTA-stat) in primary diagnosis of bladder carcinoma. Interference of blood on the results of urine-based POC tests. Anticancer Res 2012;32(5):2015–8.

24. Miyake M, Goodison S, Rizwani W, et al. Urinary BTA: indicator of bladder cancer or of hematuria. World J Urol 2012;30(6):869–73.

25. Odisho AY, Berry AB, Ahmad AE, et al. Reflex ImmunoCyt testing for the diagnosis of bladder cancer in patients with atypical urine cytology. Eur Urol 2013; 63(5):936–40.

26. Têtu B, Tiguert R, Harel F, et al. ImmunoCyt/uCyt+ improves the sensitivity of urine cytology in patients followed for urothelial carcinoma. Mod Pathol 2005; 18(1):83–9.

27. Sokolova IA, Halling KC, Jenkins RB, et al. The development of a multitarget, multicolor fluorescence in situ hybridization assay for the detection of urothelial carcinoma in urine. J Mol Diagn 2000; 2(3):116–23.

28. Hajdinjak T. UroVysion FISH test for detecting urothelial cancers: meta-analysis of diagnostic accuracy and comparison with urinary cytology testing. Urol Oncol 2008;26(6):646–51.

29. Kim PH, Sukhu R, Cordon BH, et al. Reflex fluorescence in situ hybridization assay for suspicious urinary cytology in patients with bladder cancer with negative surveillance cystoscopy. BJU Int 2014;114(3):354–9.

30. Seideman C, Canter D, Kim P, et al. Multicenter evaluation of the role of UroVysion FISH assay in surveillance of patients with bladder cancer: does FISH positivity anticipate recurrence? World J Urol 2014. http://dx.doi.org/10.1007/s00345-014-1452-9.

31. Clark SJ, Melki J. DNA methylation and gene silencing in cancer: which is the guilty party? Oncogene 2002; 21(35):5380–7.

32. Catto JW, Azzouzi AR, Rehman I, et al. Promoter hypermethylation is associated with tumor location, stage, and subsequent progression in transitional cell carcinoma. J Clin Oncol 2005;23(13):2903–10.

33. Chan MW, Chan LW, Tang NL, et al. Hypermethylation of multiple genes in tumor tissues and voided urine in urinary bladder cancer patients. Clin Cancer Res 2002;8(2):464–70.

34. Dulaimi E, Ibanez de Caceres I, Uzzo RG, et al. Promoter hypermethylation profile of kidney cancer. Clin Cancer Res 2004;10(12 Pt 1):3972–9.

35. Hoque MO, Begum S, Topaloglu O, et al. Quantitation of promoter methylation of multiple genes in urine DNA and bladder cancer detection. J Natl Cancer Inst 2006;98(14):996–1004.

36. Marsit CJ, Karagas MR, Andrew A, et al. Epigenetic inactivation of SFRP genes and TP53 alteration act jointly as markers of invasive bladder cancer. Cancer Res 2005;65(16):7081–5.

37. Yates DR, Rehman I, Abbod MF, et al. Promoter hypermethylation identifies progression risk in bladder cancer. Clin Cancer Res 2007;13(7):2046–53.

38. Yu J, Zhu T, Wang Z, et al. A novel set of DNA methylation markers in urine sediments for sensitive/specific detection of bladder cancer. Clin Cancer Res 2007; 13(24):7296–304.

39. Su SF, de Castro Abreu AL, Chihara Y, et al. A panel of three markers hyper- and hypomethylated in urine sediments accurately predicts bladder cancer recurrence. Clin Cancer Res 2014;20(7): 1978–89.

40. Kandimalla R, Masius R, Beukers W, et al. A 3-plex methylation assay combined with the FGFR3 mutation assay sensitively detects recurrent bladder

cancer in voided urine. Clin Cancer Res 2013; 19(17):4760–9.

41. Kandimalla R, van Tilborg AA, Zwarthoff EC. DNA methylation-based biomarkers in bladder cancer. Nat Rev Urol 2013;10(6):327–35.

42. Phé V, Cussenot O, Rouprêt M. Interest of methylated genes as biomarkers in urothelial cell carcinomas of the urinary tract. BJU Int 2009;104(7): 896–901.

43. Poyet C, Jentsch B, Hermanns T, et al. Expression of histone deacetylases 1, 2 and 3 in urothelial bladder cancer. BMC Clin Pathol 2014;14(1):10.

44. Li H, Wang J, Xiao W, et al. Epigenetic inactivation of KLF4 is associated with urothelial cancer progression and early recurrence. J Urol 2014;191(2):493–501.

45. Griffiths-Jones S, Grocock RJ, van Dongen S, et al. miRBase: microRNA sequences, targets and gene nomenclature. Nucleic Acids Res 2006;34:D140–4.

46. Guancial EA, Bellmunt J, Yeh S, et al. The evolving understanding of microRNA in bladder cancer. Urol Oncol 2014;32(1):41.e31–40.

47. Yoshino H, Seki N, Itesako T, et al. Aberrant expression of microRNAs in bladder cancer. Nat Rev Urol 2013;10(7):396–404.

48. Feng Y, Kang Y, He Y, et al. microRNA-99a acts as a tumor suppressor and is down-regulated in bladder cancer. BMC Urol 2014;14:50.

49. Xu C, Zeng Q, Xu W, et al. miRNA-100 inhibits human bladder urothelial carcinogenesis by directly targeting mTOR. Mol Cancer Ther 2013; 12(2):207–19.

50. Scheffer AR, Holdenrieder S, Kristiansen G, et al. Circulating microRNAs in serum: novel biomarkers for patients with bladder cancer? World J Urol 2014;32(2):353–8.

51. Eissa S, Badr S, Elhamid SA, et al. The value of combined use of survivin mRNA and matrix metalloproteinase 2 and 9 for bladder cancer detection in voided urine. Dis Markers 2013;34(1):57–62.

52. Eissa S, Badr S, Barakat M, et al. The diagnostic efficacy of urinary survivin and hyaluronidase mRNA as urine markers in patients with bladder cancer. Clin Lab 2013;59(7–8):893–900.

53. Abd El-Hakim TF, El-Shafie MK, Abdou AG, et al. Value of urinary survivin as a diagnostic marker in bladder cancer. Anal Quant Cytopathol Histpathol 2014;36(3):121–7.

54. Wang J, Zhang X, Wei P, et al. Livin, Survivin and Caspase 3 as early recurrence markers in non-muscle-invasive bladder cancer. World J Urol 2014;32(6):1477–84.

55. Burger M, Catto JW, Dalbagni G, et al. Epidemiology and risk factors of urothelial bladder cancer. Eur Urol 2013;63(2):234–41.

56. Gakis G, Efstathiou J, Lerner SP, et al. ICUD-EAU International Consultation on Bladder Cancer 2012: radical cystectomy and bladder preservation for muscle-invasive urothelial carcinoma of the bladder. Eur Urol 2013;63(1):45–57.

57. De Vivar Chevez AR, Finke J, Bukowski R. The role of inflammation in kidney cancer. Adv Exp Med Biol 2014;816:197–234.

58. Sfanos KS, Hempel HA, De Marzo AM. The role of inflammation in prostate cancer. Adv Exp Med Biol 2014;816:153–81.

59. Fitzgerald JP, Nayak B, Shanmugasundaram K, et al. Nox4 mediates renal cell carcinoma cell invasion through hypoxia-induced interleukin-6 and -8 production. PLoS One 2012;7(1):e30712.

60. Masson-Lecomte A, Rava M, Real FX, et al. Inflammatory biomarkers and bladder cancer prognosis: a systematic review. Eur Urol 2014;66:1078–91.

61. Mano R, Baniel J, Shoshany O, et al. Neutrophil-to-lymphocyte ratio predicts progression and recurrence of non-muscle-invasive bladder cancer. Urol Oncol 2014. http://dx.doi.org/10.1016/j.urolonc. 2014.06.010.

62. Van Rhijn BW. Combining molecular and pathologic data to prognosticate non-muscle-invasive bladder cancer. Urol Oncol 2012;30(4):518–23.

63. Oderda M, Ricceri F, Pisano F, et al. Prognostic factors including Ki-67 and p53 in Bacillus Calmette-Guérin-treated non-muscle-invasive bladder cancer: a prospective study. Urol Int 2013;90(2): 184–90.

64. Moonen PM, van Balken-Ory B, Kiemeney LA, et al. Prognostic value of p53 for high risk superficial bladder cancer with long-term followup. J Urol 2007;177(1):80–3.

65. Shariat SF, Ashfaq R, Sagalowsky AI, et al. Predictive value of cell cycle biomarkers in nonmuscle invasive bladder transitional cell carcinoma. J Urol 2007;177(2):481–7 [discussion: 487].

66. Castillo-Martin M, Domingo-Domenech J, Karni-Schmidt O, et al. Molecular pathways of urothelial development and bladder tumorigenesis. Urol Oncol 2010;28(4):401–8.

67. Lindgren D, Liedberg F, Andersson A, et al. Molecular characterization of early-stage bladder carcinomas by expression profiles, FGFR3 mutation status, and loss of 9q. Oncogene 2006;25(18): 2685–96.

68. Kompier LC, Lurkin I, van der Aa MN, et al. FGFR3, HRAS, KRAS, NRAS and PIK3CA mutations in bladder cancer and their potential as biomarkers for surveillance and therapy. PLoS One 2010;5(11): e13821.

69. Karam JA, Shariat SF, Hsieh JT, et al. Genomics: a preview of genomic medicine. BJU Int 2008;102(9 Pt B):1221–7.

70. Klatte T, Seligson DB, Rao JY, et al. Absent CD44v6 expression is an independent predictor of poor urothelial bladder cancer outcome. J Urol 2010;183(6): 2403–8.

71. Omran OM, Ata HS. CD44s and CD44v6 in diagnosis and prognosis of human bladder cancer. Ultrastruct Pathol 2012;36(3):145–52.

72. Shariat SF, Youssef RF, Gupta A, et al. Association of angiogenesis related markers with bladder cancer outcomes and other molecular markers. J Urol 2010;183(5):1744–50.

73. Kopparapu PK, Boorjian SA, Robinson BD, et al. Expression of VEGF and its receptors VEGFR1/VEGFR2 is associated with invasiveness of bladder cancer. Anticancer Res 2013;33(6):2381–90.

74. Huang YJ, Qi WX, He AN, et al. Prognostic value of tissue vascular endothelial growth factor expression in bladder cancer: a meta-analysis. Asian Pac J Cancer Prev 2013;14(2):645–9.

75. Siemerink MJ, Klaassen I, Vogels IM, et al. CD34 marks angiogenic tip cells in human vascular endothelial cell cultures. Angiogenesis 2012;15(1):151–63.

76. Ajili F, Kacem M, Tounsi H, et al. Prognostic impact of angiogenesis in nonmuscle invasive bladder cancer as defined by microvessel density after immunohistochemical staining for CD34. Ultrastruct Pathol 2012;36(5):336–42.

77. Kramer MW, Golshani R, Merseburger AS, et al. HYAL-1 hyaluronidase: a potential prognostic indicator for progression to muscle invasion and recurrence in bladder cancer. Eur Urol 2010;57(1):86–93.

78. Potter C, Harris AL. Hypoxia inducible carbonic anhydrase IX, marker of tumour hypoxia, survival pathway and therapy target. Cell Cycle 2004;3(2):164–7.

79. Klatte T, Seligson DB, Rao JY, et al. Carbonic anhydrase IX in bladder cancer: a diagnostic, prognostic, and therapeutic molecular marker. Cancer 2009;115(7):1448–58.

80. Yun SJ, Jo SW, Ha YS, et al. PFKFB4 as a prognostic marker in non-muscle-invasive bladder cancer. Urol Oncol 2012;30(6):893–9.

81. Klatte T, Xylinas E, Rieken M, et al. Impact of ABO blood type on outcomes in patients with primary nonmuscle invasive bladder cancer. J Urol 2014;191(5):1238–43.

82. Tilki D, Burger M, Dalbagni G, et al. Urine markers for detection and surveillance of non-muscle-invasive bladder cancer. Eur Urol 2011;60(3):484–92.

83. Yossepowitch O, Herr HW, Donat SM. Use of urinary biomarkers for bladder cancer surveillance: patient perspectives. J Urol 2007;177(4):1277–82 [discussion: 1282].

84. Bensalah K, Montorsi F, Shariat SF. Challenges of cancer biomarker profiling. Eur Urol 2007;52(6):1601–9.

85. Check E. Proteomics and cancer: running before we can walk? Nature 2004;429(6991):496–7.

86. Klatte T, Shariat SF. Novel urinary markers for detection of bladder cancer—are we failing? J Urol 2014;191(1):9–10.

87. Shariat SF, Karakiewicz PI, Ashfaq R, et al. Multiple biomarkers improve prediction of bladder cancer recurrence and mortality in patients undergoing cystectomy. Cancer 2008;112(2):315–25.

88. Gogalic S, Sauer U, Doppler S, et al. Bladder cancer biomarker array to detect aberrant levels of proteins in urine. Analyst 2015;140:724–35.

89. Todenhöfer T, Hennenlotter J, Aufderklamm S, et al. Individual risk assessment in bladder cancer patients based on a multi-marker panel. J Cancer Res Clin Oncol 2013;139(1):49–56.

90. Wang LC, Xylinas E, Kent MT, et al. Combining smoking information and molecular markers improves prognostication in patients with urothelial carcinoma of the bladder. Urol Oncol 2014;32(4):433–40.

91. Wilhelm-Benartzi CS, Koestler DC, Houseman EA, et al. DNA methylation profiles delineate etiologic heterogeneity and clinically important subgroups of bladder cancer. Carcinogenesis 2010;31(11):1972–6.

92. Cortessis VK, Yuan JM, Van Den Berg D, et al. Risk of urinary bladder cancer is associated with 8q24 variant rs9642880[T] in multiple racial/ethnic groups: results from the Los Angeles-Shanghai case-control study. Cancer Epidemiol Biomarkers Prev 2010;19(12):3150–6.

93. Gu J, Horikawa Y, Chen M, et al. Benzo(a)pyrene diol epoxide-induced chromosome 9p21 aberrations are associated with increased risk of bladder cancer. Cancer Epidemiol Biomarkers Prev 2008;17(9):2445–50.

94. Horstmann M, Todenhöfer T, Hennenlotter J, et al. Influence of age on false positive rates of urine-based tumor markers. World J Urol 2013;31(4):935–40.

95. Mengual L, Burset M, Ribal MJ, et al. Gene expression signature in urine for diagnosing and assessing aggressiveness of bladder urothelial carcinoma. Clin Cancer Res 2010;16(9):2624–33.

96. García-Baquero R, Puerta P, Beltran M, et al. Methylation of a novel panel of tumor suppressor genes in urine moves forward noninvasive diagnosis and prognosis of bladder cancer: a 2-center prospective study. J Urol 2013;190(2):723–30.

Surgical Advances in Bladder Cancer
At What Cost?

David C. Johnson, MD, MPH*, Peter S. Greene, MD,
Matthew E. Nielsen, MD, MS

KEYWORDS

- Bladder cancer • Alvimopan • Blue-light cystoscopy • Robotic cystectomy • Costs • Quality of life

KEY POINTS

- Bladder cancer is one of the most expensive cancers to treat; however, funding for research, discovery, and innovation is relatively lacking.
- Blue-light cystoscopy is a novel diagnostic and therapeutic technique that improves detection of superficial bladder cancer and reduces costs associated with tumor recurrence.
- Alvimopan, an oral opioid receptor antagonist, reduces the incidence and costs of complications associated with postoperative ileus after radical cystectomy and small bowel urinary diversion.
- Robot-assisted radical cystectomy is an oncologically acceptable alternative to open cystectomy; however, further investigation is necessary to determine the cost-effectiveness of this technology.

INTRODUCTION

From diagnosis to death, bladder cancer is the most expensive malignancy to treat in the United States, with estimated expenditures of up to $187,000 per incident case.[1,2] Bladder cancer treatment accounted for approximately $4 billion in direct costs to the US health care system in 2010 and is expected to exceed $5 billion by 2020.[3]

Direct costs related to the management of non-muscle invasive bladder cancer (NMIBC) are driven by regular surveillance cystoscopies, frequent cross-sectional imaging and repetitive transurethral resections of bladder tumors (TURBT), and intravesical therapies.[4–6] Patients typically have prolonged survival with frequent recurrences resulting in the high lifetime cost of this disease. Given that approximately 75% of incident cases are in this subgroup, the potential economic and public health impact of innovation in NMIBC is substantial.

For patients with muscle-invasive bladder cancer (MIBC), the standard of care is radical cystectomy (RC) with bilateral pelvic lymph node dissection and urinary diversion.[4–6] Despite improvements in surgical techniques and postoperative recovery pathways, this complex and challenging procedure remains highly morbid with up to 60% of patients experiencing a complication[7–9] and 25% requiring readmission to the hospital within 30 days.[10] In addition to the high cost of surgery and management of subsequent complications, perioperative chemotherapy, and frequent cross-sectional surveillance imaging, as well as high end-of-life costs, contribute to the substantial financial burden of advanced disease.[11] In addition to the direct medical costs associated with health services expenditures, the societal value of life lost because of untimely death from bladder cancer in the year 2000 alone is estimated to be as high as $17 billion.[12]

Department of Urology, University of North Carolina, School of Medicine, 2113 Physician's Office Building, 170 Manning Drive, CB 7235, Chapel Hill, NC 27599, USA
* Corresponding author.
E-mail address: David.Johnson3@unchealth.unc.edu

Urol Clin N Am 42 (2015) 235–252
http://dx.doi.org/10.1016/j.ucl.2015.01.005

Surgical advancements and novel diagnostic and therapeutic techniques are essential to improve bladder cancer outcomes and reduce the burden of suffering. However, the cost-effectiveness of these advances has never been more relevant as pressure mounts on the health care system to contain costs. Bladder cancer represents an enormous opportunity to maximize the value of treatment to improve outcomes while reducing excessive expenditures.[13] This article examines the effectiveness and costs associated with recent advances in the surgical management of bladder cancer. In the first section, the evidence regarding blue light cystoscopy as an innovation in NMIBC is discussed; subsequently, with regard to patient care for higher risk disease, the novel perioperative pharmaceutical, alvimopam, and robotic-assisted radical cystectomy (RARC) are evaluated.

BLUE-LIGHT CYSTOSCOPY
Rationale

Complete TURBT is paramount to optimizing oncologic outcomes and minimizing costs.[14] Approximately 60% of patients with newly diagnosed NMIBC have an "early recurrence" within 1 year after initial TURBT.[15] Because nearly one-third of patients undergoing repeat TURBT within 6 weeks of initial resection have residual tumor, a substantial proportion of these recurrences may represent incomplete initial resection.[16] Although solitary, pedunculated, papillary lesions are adequately visualized and resected with traditional white-light cystoscopy (WLC), the risk of incomplete detection and/or tumor resection with WLC is particularly high with flat, sessile, multifocal lesions characteristic of carcinoma in situ (CIS).[17–19] Intravesical therapies are intended to treat and prevent implantation of microscopic tumor cells rather than gross residual tumor burden. Recurrence, progression, and overall prognosis are therefore strongly predicated on the completeness of the initial TURBT.

Description

Blue-light cystoscopy (BLC) or fluorescence cystoscopy was developed to improve detection to increase the likelihood of complete TURBT. This optical-imaging technology uses a photosensitizing agent in combination with blue-light illumination (380–450 nm) to help differentiate between malignant and benign urothelium. The photosensitizing agent is actively transported into urothelial cytoplasm and incorporated by the cellular heme-biosynthesis metabolism. The photoactive component (photoporphyrin IV) accumulates in cancerous and precancerous cells as a result of abnormal enzyme activity, while normal tissue eliminates the photoactive substance. When illuminated by blue light, abnormal cells fluoresce red from the accumulation of photoporphyrins and are more easily differentiated from the bluish-green appearance of normal cells.[20]

The original photosensitizing agent, 5-amnolevulinic acid (5-ALA), required a 2- to 4-hour intravesical dwell time before TURBT and is no longer commercially available. Hexaminolevulinate (HAL; Cysview, PhotoCure Inc, Princeton, NJ, USA; formerly Hexvix, Photocure ASA, Oslo, Norway) is a derivative of 5-ALA that was approved for use in Europe in 2006 and in the United States in 2010.[21] HAL and 5-ALA are equally effective[22]; however, HAL is more stable in white light, has better fluorescent intensity, has more homogeneous enhancement and distribution within photoactive porphyrins, and requires only 1 hour of dwell time.[23]

Efficacy

Literature summary
Two meta-analyses by were published in 2013 by Yuan and colleagues[24] (12 articles from 11 studies, 2258 patients, 1114 receiving BLC, including patients receiving 5-ALA and HAL) and Burger and colleagues[18] (10 articles from 9 studies, 2212 patients, 1345 receiving BLC, only HAL). The meta-analysis by Burger and colleagues used raw patient-level data from prospective studies of patients receiving only HAL and provides the strongest level of evidence for the benefit of BLC. Rink and colleagues[25] also published a systematic review of 44 studies comparing both 5-ALA and HAL with WLC in 2013.

Increased detection
Ta/T1 Burger and colleagues[18] demonstrated significant improvement in the detection of papillary lesions with BLC using HAL (95% vs 86%, odds ratio [OR] 4.9 P<.0001). The odds of detecting a T1 lesion were 2.3 times higher with BLC than with WLC. One in 4 patients had at least 1 additional tumor detected by BLC that was missed with WLC in this meta-analysis. This proportion of patients with a missed tumor on WLC detected by BLC was significant in both primary (20.7%) and recurrent (27.7%) disease as well as intermediate-risk (35.7%) and high-risk (27.0%) disease. The detection rate in studies reviewed by Rink and colleagues[25] using BLC was 92% to 100% compared with 50% to 100% using WLC.

Carcinoma in situ The odds of detecting CIS was 12.4 times higher with BLC than WLC (95% vs 59%, P<.0001) with 26.7% of patients having

CIS detected only by BLC.[18] Detection rates for CIS ranged from 49% to 100% with BLC and 5% to 68% with WLC in studies reviewed by Rink and colleagues.[25]

Recurrence

Both meta-analyses demonstrated decreased risk of recurrence with BLC. Yuan and colleagues[24] reported that BLC reduced recurrence from 47.8% to 32.7% (OR 0.5, 95% confidence interval [CI] 0.4–0.6; $P<.00001$). Burger and colleagues[18] reported the recurrence was reduced from 45.4% to 34.5% with BLC (OR 0.8, 95% CI 0.6–0.9; $P = .006$). BLC was slightly more effective in reducing recurrences of CIS or T1 tumors (OR 0.7, $P = .05$) compared with Ta disease (0.8, $P = .04$). In this meta-analysis, the number needed to treat with BLC to avoid 1 tumor recurrence was 6. The time to first recurrence was 1.7 months longer with BLC than WLC (95% CI 0.9–2.5 months; $P<.0001$).

Progression-free survival

No difference in progression-free survival (PFS) was noted at 1 year. In studies reviewed by Rink and colleagues,[25] PFS ranged from 89% to 98% with BLC and 89% to 95% with WLC. Yuan and colleagues[24] also reported no difference in PFS (OR 0.9, 95% CI 0.6–1.2, $P = .39$). Because of the natural history of NMIBC, measuring PFS at 1 year may be too short of a follow-up period to evaluate the impact of BLC on this intermediate outcome.

Safety

No safety concerns were discovered in an evaluation of more than 2300 patients who received HAL with BLC in 6 controlled trials.[26] No serious adverse events (SAEs) or deaths were definitively attributed to administration of HAL, while 8 SAEs in 6 patients were of uncertain relationship to HAL. Adverse events (AEs) leading to treatment discontinuation occurred in 0.8% of all patients who received HAL compared with 0.2% who only underwent WLC. Only 2 AEs in one patient had uncertain relationship to HAL. There was no increased toxicity with dwell time exceeding 1 hour and no apparent drug-drug, drug-food, or drug-disease interactions. Finally, no significant increase in AEs or anaphylactic reactions was identified with repeated use of HAL within a controlled trial setting or on postmarketing evaluation of greater than 200,000 procedures from 2004 to 2013, where 23% received HAL more than once and 8% received HAL more than twice.[26] Nevertheless, the US Food and Drug Administration (FDA) approval remains limited to one-time dose due to a single anaphylactic event after repeat administration that was not clearly related to HAL.[27]

Guidelines and Recommendations

The European Association of Urology (EAU) recommends using BLC with HAL at initial TURBT.[6] Although the International Consortium of Urologic Diseases (ICUD) suggests BLC improves tumor detection on initial TURBT, particularly with CIS, they make no definitive statement recommending routine use.[18] The last iteration of the American Urological Association guidelines on NMIBC was completed before FDA approval of HAL and therefore offers no guidance.[4] Several additional European and North American expert consensus groups echo the EAU recommendation for use on initial resection.[19,28,29] Expert consensus statements from Europe[19] and the United States[30] recommend using BLC in several additional settings, as shown in **Table 1**.

Cost Analysis

Several European studies[14,31–34] and one from the United States[35] report cost comparison analyses with BLC and WLC. Additional expenditures with BLC included costs of the photodynamic medication, Foley catheters for instillation, increased surveillance cystoscopies for patients upstaged to high risk by BLC, and capital investment in BLC-compatible endoscopic equipment. Cost savings were primarily derived from fewer TURBTs. The studies varied slightly in their cost assumptions and duration of follow-up included in the analysis, as shown in **Table 2**.

Utility/Quality of Life

To the extent that BLC reduces recurrences and the need for associated TURBTs, this technology is likely to improve patient quality of life (QOL), as suggested by Malmstrom and colleagues and Grossman and colleagues.[34,36] To date, however, empirical data on the effect of BLC on QOL are limited.

Using statistical modeling based on clinical trials data, Marteau and colleagues[37] estimated that patients receiving BLC spend 11% less time managing recurrences over a period of 5 years. In the absence of empirically derived utility scores for the relevant clinical states in the model, the actual effect on QOL remains somewhat speculative, but the concept of a QOL benefit associated with a reduction in recurrences and procedures required to manage these has face validity. Further research to elucidate the clinically relevant benefit of BLC on QOL is necessary.

Table 1
Guidelines and expert consensus statements on the use of blue-light cystoscopy

Setting	Bladder Cancer Guidelines (BCG)		Expert Consensus Statements	
	EAU 2013[6] (Babjuk)	ICUD-EAU 2013[18] (Burger)	USA 2014[30] (Daneshmand)	European 2014[19] (Witjes)
Initial TURBT	+	n/a	+	+
Positive cytology and negative WLC	n/a	+	+	+
Aid in diagnosis of CIS	+	+	+	+
Assess for suspected tumor recurrence	n/a	n/a	+	(+)
Follow-up of patients at intermediate to high risk of recurrence (high-grade T1, CIS, multifocal tumors)	n/a	n/a	+	+
In patients having received intravesical therapy (BCG)	n/a	n/a	+[a]	(+)[b]
In patients having repeat TURBT within 6 wk	n/a	n/a	+	(+)
Surveillance office cystoscopy or cystoscopy for hematuria workup	−	−	n/a	−
As a training tool	−	−	n/a	+
Repeat TURBT in patients with high risk of recurrence who had prior TURBT with BLC	n/a	n/a	n/a	(+)

+, recommended; (+), recommended with proviso; −, insufficient data to recommend or not recommend; n/a, not reported.
[a] At least 3 mo after BCG.
[b] At least 6 wk after BCG.
Data from Refs. 6,18,19,30

Gaps in Knowledge and Further Research

Variation in the utilization of perioperative single-dose intravesical chemotherapy is a major confounder across the studies evaluating BLC. Only 45% of patients in the phase III North American trial received single-dose chemotherapy, and it was not administered systematically. O'Brien and colleagues[38] found no recurrence reduction with BLC over a period of 1 year in 168 patients. However, despite attempting to administer single-dose mitomycin C (MMC) systematically, only 63% of patients undergoing BLC and 77% of patients undergoing WLC actually received the chemotherapy. Geavlete and colleagues,[39] conversely, found a significant reduction in recurrence with BLC over a period of 2 years when all 239 patients in their study received single-dose MMC.

To address this limitation of the existing literature, the PHOTOdynamic trial recently opened in the United Kingdom (http://www.controlled-trials.com/ISRCTN84013636). This trial plans to randomize 533 patients with newly diagnosed bladder cancer to BLC or WLC on initial TURBT, with systematic administration of perioperative intravesical chemotherapy, standardized risk-adjusted surveillance protocol, and appropriate adjuvant therapies.

ROBOT-ASSISTED LAPAROSCOPIC RADICAL CYSTECTOMY
Introduction

In the context of treatment of patients with more advanced disease, minimally invasive approaches to RC with pelvic lymph node dissection were developed in hopes of reducing the substantial morbidity of one of the most technical and challenging operations performed by urologists. Menon and colleagues[40] described the first report of the RARC in 2003. Utilization of this technology for extirpative bladder surgery has subsequently risen to more than 12% as of 2011.[41,42] Given trends in the adoption of robotic prostatectomy, it is possible that a continued increase in the utilization of RARC may be seen because trainees are more frequently getting experience with RARC in residency, and an increasing number of practicing urologists become more comfortable with robotics through experience with prostate and kidney surgery. As with many surgical innovations, adoption of RARC has preceded rigorous outcome and cost-effectiveness analyses.

Safety and Oncologic Efficacy

Three systematic reviews with meta-analyses compare complications and surrogate markers of oncologic efficacy (soft tissue margin positivity rate and lymph node yield) between open radical cystectomy (ORC) and RARC.[43–45] With only one prospective randomized trial included available for review,[46] these analyses suffer from inclusion of primarily small, single-center retrospective studies with inherent selection biases.

In general, these reviews conclude that RARC is associated with lower complications, less blood loss, fewer blood transfusions, shorter length of stay (LOS), but longer operative times. Three additional small, nonrandomized studies[47–49] and a propensity-matched population-based cohort study[41] subsequently confirmed these findings.

Patients undergoing RARC have a favorable positive surgical margin rate and lymph node yield compared with ORC.[43–45] A subsequent propensity matched cohort study supported these findings by demonstrating a higher overall lymph node yield and lower positive soft tissue margin rate.[50]

Recognizing the inherent limitations of available data, RARC appears feasible and safe with satisfactory oncologic outcomes. In 2013, however, the EAU stated that they were unable to form definite conclusions regarding the long-term safety and efficacy of RARC because of the lack of high-level evidence and long-term follow-up.[51]

Two subsequent prospective randomized trials comparing safety and oncologic outcomes between ORC and RARC were recently published,[52,53] adding to the findings of the randomized controlled trial by Nix and colleagues[46] in 2010 (**Table 3**). The RAZOR multicenter randomized trial has completed accrual of 350 patients, with follow-up ongoing, and will provide more definitive high-level evidence in the near future.

There is a relative paucity of high-quality long-term oncologic outcome data due to the relatively recent adoption of RARC.[54] Two recent single-institution, retrospective analyses of the earliest RARC cohorts with 5- to 8-year follow-up suggest long-term oncologic outcomes comparable to ORC series, including overall, disease-specific, and disease-free survival.[55,56] Prospective randomized controlled trials with long-term follow-up are necessary before making definitive conclusions about the safety and efficacy of RARC; however, preliminary data suggest similar outcomes.

Costs

Current cost assessments of RARC and ORC are limited to cost-identification analyses, which assume equivalent outcomes with both techniques. Long-term functional and oncologic outcomes are still maturing and have yet to be integrated

Table 2
Cost analyses of blue-light cystoscopy

Study	Cost Savings in $/Person (Time Frame)	Assumptions/Oncologic Outcomes	Notes
Dindyal et al,[31] 2008	712 (first year)	20% reduction in recurrence at 3 mo 20% fewer TURBTs 20% fewer doses of MMC 30% reduction in surveillance cystoscopies per year	New cases of NMIBC in the UK Standardized HRG costs for TURBT, MMC, cystoscopy Uses 5-ALA for analysis
Sievert et al,[14] 2009	173 (first 3–6 mo)	20% reduction in recurrence at 3 mo 20% fewer TURBTs	New cases of NMIBC in Germany at single institution Includes costs of preoperative catheter and HAL, additional equipment costs for BLC amortised over 10 y, equipment and staffing costs for TURBT, pathology costs
Burger et al,[32] 2007	208 (per year for 7 y)	None, compared actual treatment and follow-up treatment costs in randomized cohort 60% fewer TURBTs per person (0.8 vs 2.0 per person in BLC vs WLC group)	Patients randomized to WLC or BLC in single German center All patients with NMIBC underwent repeat TURBT at prior resection site after 6 wk, appropriate adjuvant intravesical therapy, and quarterly surveillance cystoscopy Mean follow-up of 7.1 y Included single additional expenditure for each patient receiving BLC to account for medication (5-ALA) and catheter Identical rates of progression to MIBC so these costs not analyzed

Study	Cost	Outcomes	Comments
Otto et al,[33] 2009	Low risk: 209 (per year for 8.3 y) Intermediate risk: 335 (per year for 8.3 y) High risk: 259 (per year for 8.3 y)	Lower recurrence rate in BLC group (28 vs 57%)	Long-term (8.3 y) follow-up of Burger et al, 2007 Separated cost analysis into risk subgroups
Malstrom et al,[34] 2009	83 (first year)	40% reduction in recurrences 7% reduction in need for TURBT 1% reduction in surveillance cystoscopy 44% reduction in cystectomy	Population-based modeling estimate of first-year cost saving to the Swedish health care system based on 2032 new bladder cancer cases Included costs of cystoscopy, TURBT, post-TURBT treatments (MMC and/or BCG for NMIBC, cystectomy, and/or chemotherapy for MIBC or metastatic disease)
Garfield et al,[35] 2013	932 (first year)	Model derived from incidence, recurrence, and progression rates as well as rates of treatment of MIBC from long-term follow-up of original clinical trial by Stenzl et al (Grossman, 2012) Tumor-free rate (31.8 vs 38% in WLC vs BLC groups) Median time to recurrence (9.6 vs 16.4 mo in WLC vs BLC groups) Overall development of MIBC (6.1 vs 3.1% in WLC vs BLC groups) Cystectomy for progression (7.9 vs 4.8% in WLC vs BLC groups)	Probabilistic decision-tree model for overall US health care system costs using HAL BLC at initial diagnosis as adjunct to WLC over 5 y Did not take costs of capital equipment into account because modeling was from the perspective of reimbursement by payers Used median Medicare payment

Abbreviation: HRG, Healthcare Resource Group.
Data from Refs.[14,31–35]

Table 3
Randomized controlled trials comparing perioperative outcomes and oncologic efficiency between RARC and ORC

Authors	Study Characteristics	Complications (RARC vs ORC)	Perioperative Factors (RARC vs ORC)	Oncologic Efficacy (RARC vs ORC)
Nix et al,[46] 2010	Prospective single-center noninferiority RCT N = 41 (RARC = 21, ORC = 20)	Any complication: 33 vs 50% Total Clavien units: 1.7 vs 2.8 (P = .05)	OR time: 4.2 vs 3.5 h (P<.0001) EBL: 274 vs 564 mL (P = .0003) Time to BM: 3.2 vs 4.3 d (P = .0003) In-house analgesia; 93.6 vs 151.6 mg (P = .01) LOS 5.4 vs 6 d (P = .42)	LN yield: equivalent (18 vs 19, P = .5)
Parekh et al,[52] 2013	Pilot prospective single center RCT N = 39 (RARC = 20, ORC = 19)	Clavien 2 or greater: 25 vs 25% (P = .5)	OR time: 5.0 vs 4.75 h (P = .33) EBL: 400 vs 800 mL (0.003) Transfusions (40 vs 50%, P = .27) LOS: 6 vs 6 d (P = .29) LOS 5 d or less (35% vs 10%, P = .03) Days to diet: 4 vs 5.5 d (P = .5)	LN yield: equivalent 11 vs 23 (P = .135) PSM: 5 vs 5% (P = .5)
Bochner et al,[53] 2014	Prospective single-center RCT N = 118 (RARC = 58, ORC = 60	Clavien 2–5: 62 vs 66% (P = .66) Clavien 3–5: 22 vs 21% (P = .9)	OR time: 7.6 vs 5.5 h (P<.001) EBL: 159 mL less with RARC LOS: 8 vs 8 d (P = .53)	n/a

Abbreviations: BM, bowel movement; EBL, estimated blood loss; LN, lymph node; OR, operating room; PSM, positive surgical margins; RARC, robot-assisted radical cystectomy; RCT, randomized control trial.
Data from Refs.[46,52,53]

into proper cost-effectiveness analyses using quality-adjusted life years (QALY). Additional challenges to effective cost assessments are the variable structure of robotic equipment purchases and maintenance, different operating room and hospitalization costs between institutions, and heterogeneous robotic operative experience.

Generally speaking, existing cost analyses of RARC account for additional direct fixed costs (initial robot purchase, maintenance, disposable instruments) and direct variable costs (operating room time) with indirect cost savings associated with reduced blood loss, fewer transfusions, avoidance of complications, shorter LOS, and decreased medication requirement. Additional theoretic cost benefits that have yet to be quantified in this particular context include faster convalescence with a reduction in lost productivity. Three single-institutional cost analyses have been performed with somewhat mixed results.[57–59] These studies consider the direct and indirect costs mentioned above (**Table 4**). The lack of long-term follow-up and clinical outcomes thus far limits the assessment of long-term costs.[60]

Two additional population-based cohort analyses evaluated the cost difference between RARC and ORC in the United States using the National Inpatient Sample[61] and the Premier Perspective Database,[41] an all-payer hospital discharge database. Yu and colleagues[61] concluded that the robotic approach adds an additional $3797 per case and Leow and colleagues[41] estimated an additional per case cost of $4236, primarily because of increased supply costs. An additional important finding is that the cost difference disappears in high-volume centers (≥ 19 cases per year) or if performed by a high-volume surgeon (≥ 7 cases per year).[41]

Conclusion

Although lacking the ability to perform the preferred cost per QALY analysis, RARC has been consistently associated with increased direct fixed costs of equipment purchase, maintenance, and the use of expensive disposable instruments. However, as robot ownership becomes increasingly ubiquitous with greater utilization for prostatectomy, partial nephrectomy, and gynecologic and general surgery procedures, additional equipment costs for RARC may be effectively marginalized, particularly in relatively higher volume facilities. In addition, with greater operative experience and increased centralization of RARC in high-volume centers, variable costs associated with additional operating room times may continue to

decrease. Studies already suggest the indirect cost benefit of RARC with regards to blood loss, transfusion requirement, medication and supplemental nutrition use, and LOS. Synthesizing costs with health care utilities is the essential next, albeit challenging, step.

Quality of Life

Prior postcystectomy QOL analyses demonstrated a return to baseline functional status after approximately 12 months following ORC.[62,63] Although 3 studies measuring post-RARC QOL suggest faster return to baseline function,[61,64,65] direct comparisons to ORC reveal minimal differences in postoperative QOL measures (**Table 5**).[66,67]

Larger, prospective randomized studies such as the RAZOR trial with longer follow-up are needed to make definitive conclusions on how the surgical approach affects QOL after cystectomy.[68]

ALVIMOPAN
Description

Postoperative LOS is an important factor affecting both patient experience and costs of bladder cancer care, and postoperative ileus (POI) is the most common complication affecting this variable for cystectomy. Approximately 15% of patients develop a POI at RC, which increases the risk of additional cardiovascular (CV), pulmonary, thromboembolic, and wound complications through nausea, vomiting, aspiration, abdominal distention, malnutrition, and prolonged immobility.[7,69–73] μ-Opioid receptor antagonists have emerged as a potentially useful and cost-effective adjunct to expedite convalescence after RC. Alvimopan (Entereg; Cubist Pharmaceuticals, Inc, Lexington, MA, USA) is an oral, peripherally acting μ-opioid receptor antagonist that binds with high affinity and selectivity to μ-opioid receptors in the gastrointestinal tract. At clinically appropriate doses, the large molecular size and high polarity of alvimopan limit passage into the central nervous system and therefore do not diminish the efficacy of centrally acting μ-opioid analgesics.[74] Alvimopan (12 mg oral tablet) is typically administered between 30 minutes and 5 hours before surgery, then twice daily starting the day after surgery for up to 7 days. No more than 15 doses are recommended because of a slight increase in CV events with chronic use. Alvimopan is contraindicated in patients who have taken therapeutic doses of opioids for more than 7 consecutive days before surgery, and those with severe hepatic impairment or end-stage renal disease.[75]

Table 4
Cost-identification analysis of RARC compared with open radical cystectomy

Authors	Direct Equipment Difference ($/%)	Variable Cost Difference ($/%)	Overall Cost Difference ($/%)	Assumptions
Smith et al,[57] 2010	(+)$1634	OR costs: (+)$570 Transfusions, LOS: (−)$564	(+)1640	5 y amortization 288 cases per year Equivalent complications and LOS
Martin et al,[58] 2011	(+)16%	Hospitalization costs: (−)60%	(−)38%	7 y amortization, 300 cases per year Shorter OR time with RARC (280 vs 320 min) Shorter LOS with RARC (5 vs 10 d)
Lee et al,[59] 2011[a]	IC: (+)4% CCD: (+)0.06% ON: (+)10%	IC: (−)77% CCD: (−)24% ON: (+)12%	IC: (−)19% CCD: (−)3% ON: (+)10%	7 y amortization OR time similar Shorter LOS with RARC (5.5 vs 8 d) Shorter LOS due to complications with RARC (3.1 vs 6.2 d)

Abbreviations: CCD, continent cutaneous diversion; IC, ileal conduit; ON, orthotopic neobladder; OR, operating room.
[a] Evaluated different diversion types.
Data from Refs.[57–59]

Table 5
Studies on quality of life after robot-assisted radical cystectomy and comparing quality of life after robotic-assisted or open radical cystectomy

Study	Study Characteristics	QOL Instrument	Results
Yu et al,[61] 2012	34 patients Single institution Prospective analysis RARC only	FACT-BL Preoperative baseline Every 3 mo postoperatively	Physical well-being: return to preoperative baseline by 6 mo Social/family well-being: no change Functional well-being: return to preoperative baseline by 6 mo Emotional well-being: increase from preoperative baseline Bladder-cancer-specific domains: increase from preoperative baseline by 6 mo
Stegemann et al,[64] 2012	91 patients Single institution Prospective analysis RARC only Intracorporeal and extracorporeal diversions	CDI: difference between baseline CARE and day 7 postoperative CARE score Preoperative baseline, 7 d postoperatively, up to 90 d postoperatively	Time to recover 90% of the CDI • Overall: 63 d • Pain: 33 d • Cognition: 57 d • Activity: 82 d • GI function: did not reach in 90 d
Poch et al,[65] 2014	43 patients Single institution Prospective analysis RARC only	BCI EORTC BIS	Urinary domain: return to baseline by 1–2 mo Bowel domain: return to baseline by 2–4 mo Sexual domain: return to baseline by 16–24 mo BIS: return to baseline by 10 mo
Messer et al,[66] 2014	40 patients Prospective RCT ORC vs RARC	Functional Assessment of Cancer Therapy–Vanderbilt Cystectomy Index Preoperative, every 3 mo to 1 y	No significant difference in social/family, emotional, or functional well-being at baseline, 3, 6, 9, or 12 mo Slight improvement in physical well-being with RARC at 6 mo, otherwise no significant difference at other time points
Aboumohamed et al,[67] 2014	182 patients Multi-institutional retrospective analysis ORC vs RARC	BCI EORTC BIS Preoperatively, 6 wk postoperatively, every 3 mo for 1 y, then every 6 mo	No significant difference in urinary ($P = .11$), bowel ($P = .58$), or body image ($P = .93$) Slight improvement in sexual function in ORC group ($P = .047$)

Abbreviations: BCI, Bladder Cancer Index; BIS, Body Image Scale; CARE, convalescence and recovery evaluation; CDI, CARE difference index; EORTC, European Organization for Research and Treatment of Cancer; FACT-BL, functional assessment of cancer therapy-bladder cancer; GI, gastrointestinal; RCT, randomized control trial.
Data from Refs.[61,64–67]

No significant AEs are associated with alvimopan and a 2008 *Cochrane Review* concluded that alvimopan has an equivalent safety profile to placebo.[76]

Efficacy

General surgery literature

Much of the initial experience with Alvimopan accrued in the general surgery context. Alvimopan administration resulted in shorter time to recovery of gastrointestinal function and shorter LOS after abdominal surgery in 5 randomized controlled trials.[77–81] A 2008 *Cochrane Review* subsequently concluded that alvimopan was effective in reversing opioid-induced increased gastrointestinal transit time and constipation.[76] Based on the results of these randomized trials, the FDA approved alvimopan in 2008 for prevention of POI.

However, the predominance of large-bowel resection in these studies limits extrapolation to the RC population, where small bowel resection (SBR) is more commonplace. SBR was performed in only 5% to 12% of patients in 3 of the studies[77,80,81]; one study did not specify the proportion of SBR patients,[79] and no patients underwent SBR in one of the studies.[78]

Urologic literature

Since the approval of alvimopan in 2008, significant progress has been made in defining early recovery clinical care pathways after RC to reduce the incidence and adverse effects of POI. Alvimopan, however, is not included in most pathways given the lack of evidence in patients undergoing RC.[82–85]

A small, nonrandomized, noncontrolled study of patients undergoing cystectomy with and without alvimopan was published by Vora and colleagues[86] in 2014. Of 80 patients who underwent cystectomy from 2008 to 2012 at 2 institutions, 42 received alvimopan and 38 did not. Primary results included return of bowel function, initiation of diet, LOS, and gastrointestinal complications. Patients who received alvimopan had significantly shorter time to first flatus (3.1 vs 4.7 days) and first bowel movement (3.9 vs 4.9 days), earlier initiation of clear liquid (4.1 vs 5.5 days) and regular diets (5.2 vs 6.3 days), and shorter LOS (6.1 vs 7.7 days). Surprisingly, not a single patient who received alvimopan had a prolonged POI, as compared with 26.2% of patients who did not receive alvimopan. This study is limited by its nonrandomized, non-placebo-controlled, nonblinded design as well as its small size.

A multicenter randomized, placebo-controlled trial comparing clinical outcomes with and without alvimopan in patients undergoing RC for bladder cancer was recently published by Lee and colleagues.[87] A total of 264 patients were randomized and completed the trial (n = 137 randomized to alvimopan; n = 127 randomized to placebo). Return of bowel function was the primary outcome in this study and occurred significantly faster in the study group (5.5 vs 6.8 days). Other secondary outcomes, including time to discharge order being placed (6.9 vs 7.8 days) and postoperative LOS (7.44 vs 10.07 days), favored the alvimopan group. Patients receiving alvimopan also had significantly decreased risk of prolonged LOS greater than 7 day (32.9 vs 51.5%), overall POI-related morbidity (8.4 vs 29.1%), nasogastric tube insertion (7.7 vs 24.6%), and prolonged LOS due to POI (3.5 vs 21.8%). There was no difference in readmission rate or overall incidence of AEs requiring treatment. The incidence of SAEs was lower in the alvimopan group compared with placebo (25.7 vs 48.9%). Predetermined and systematically collected CV outcomes, including CV death, myocardial infarction, unstable angina, cerebrovascular accident, congestive heart failure, serious arrhythmia, and cardiac arrest, were no different between groups. Based on the results of this randomized trial, the FDA expanded its indication to include patients undergoing bowel resection in the setting of RC in October 2013.

Cost

The published wholesale price of alvimopan 12 mg capsule is $62.50. The median number of doses administered in the aforementioned randomized trials was between 9 and 10, resulting in a total drug cost ranging from $562.50 to $625, with a maximum cost of $937.50 for all 15 doses.[88]

General surgery literature

Bell and colleagues[89] performed a post-hoc cost analysis of the 4 original North American phase III clinical trials[77–80] and concluded that routine administration of alvimopan resulted in cost savings of $879 to $977 per patient.

Additional reports with varying study populations and designs all demonstrated significant cost savings with routine alvimopan use in patients undergoing major abdominal surgery with bowel resection (**Table 6**).

Urologic literature

Hilton and colleagues[93] performed a decision-tree cost-effectiveness analysis model comparing routine use of alvimopan in RC patients to no alvimopan. The authors concluded that routine alvimopan was cost-effective assuming a baseline POI rate of 15.6% (from published literature), a 50% lower risk of POI with alvimopan, a 4-day

Table 6
Cost analysis of alvimopan in patients undergoing major abdominal surgery with bowel resection

	Cost Savings ($/patient)	Study Design	Notes
Poston et al,[90] 2011	1040	Retrospective matched cohort Large, national, in-hospital, patient-level administrative database (Premier Perspective Database)	Due primarily to decreased LOS (~1 d) with alvimopan Similar POI-related and overall morbidity
Delany et al,[91] 2012	2345 (overall) 1382 (laparoscopic) 3218 (open)	Retrospective matched cohort Large, national, in-hospital, patient-level administrative database (Premier Perspective Database)	Alvimopan significantly decreased POI-related, GI, and CV morbidity, ICU time, and LOS (~1 d)
Touchette et al,[92] 2012	2021	Formal decision model based on published clinical trial data	Assumed shorter LOS of 18.4 h with an average of 9.5 doses of alvimopan

Abbreviations: GI, gastrointestinal; ICU, intensive care unit; POI, postoperative ileus.
Data from Refs.[90–92]

increase in LOS with POI, and a drug cost of $700 per person. A sensitivity analysis revealed that alvimopan resulted in cost savings provided POI increased LOS by at least 3.5 days; the rate of POI was at least 14%, and alvimopan reduced POI by at least 44%. Robust probabilistic sensitivity analyses were performed concluding a high (74.2%) likelihood of cost saving under the given assumptions. This analysis, however, was restricted to direct costs, did not address additional indirect cost savings by shorter LOS and decreased POI, and therefore, may underestimate the true benefit of alvimopan.

Kauf and colleagues[94] reported a cost-consequence analysis using prospectively collected resource utilization data from the recently published phase IV efficacy trial[87] to compare direct POI-related costs as well as total combined costs between patients who routinely received alvimopan and placebo. The authors concluded that alvimopan significantly reduced per patient POI-related hospitalization and follow-up costs by $2340. In this study, cost savings due to shorter LOS (2.6 days) and decreased utilization of gastrointestinal-related medications and parenteral nutrition more than offset the $822 per patient medication cost in the alvimopan cohort.

Conclusion

Alvimopan, a μ-opioid antagonist, improves postoperative bowel motility and reduces the risk of POI and prolonged LOS in randomized trials of general surgery and urology patients undergoing bowel resection. Although indirect cost savings

have yet to be elucidated, routine use of alvimopan appears to reduce direct costs by decreasing expenditures on prolonged LOS, POI management, and associated complications. Data on indirect costs and QOL are sparse, but likely favor the use of alvimopan and warrant further investigation. Routine use of perioperative alvimopan in patients undergoing RC appears to be a high-value adjunct to existing clinical care pathways promoting early recovery after an expensive and morbid procedure.

SUMMARY

Given the large and growing clinical and financial burden of bladder cancer, surgical advances and novel diagnostic and therapeutic techniques are desperately needed. Although prostate and kidney cancer mortality have decreased by 17% and 14%, respectively, since the 1980s, bladder cancer mortality has improved by a mere 1%.[95] On a per-patient basis, the clinical management of bladder cancer continues to be the most expensive cancer site from diagnosis to death; progress in this context is hindered by the fact that bladder cancer also receives the lowest amount of research funding dollars per incident case.[96,97]

NMIBC represents the overwhelming majority of incident and prevalent bladder cancer cases and is characterized by the highest recurrence rate of any cancer site. Against this backdrop, the advent of fluorescence cystoscopy may represent an innovation with the potential for substantial public health and economic impact. Although additional evidence is needed to demonstrate a reduction in progression risk, the preponderance of data supports a reduced recurrence risk, which alone may be associated with substantial positive impact.

Among the subgroup of patients with higher risk disease, although RC with intestinal urinary diversion is recommended where practical, the potential morbidity and associated costs of this procedure are profound. RARC and alvimopan have emerged as 2 approaches with the potential to mitigate these risks. Although the existing literature consistently supports the favorable combination of reduced costs and improved outcomes for alvimopan, the outcomes and economics of RARC are less clear. In high-volume, experienced centers, the cost/benefit balance seems consistently favorable, but the picture is decidedly less clear among centers with less experience and lower volume.

A fundamental limitation of the current literature on patient-centered cost-effectiveness for emerging technologies in this space is the relative paucity of empirically derived data on utilities and other measures directly quantifying the QOL impact of different clinical states in bladder cancer survivorship.[98] Furthermore, variable cost perspectives (patient, hospital, payer, health system), interinstitutional variations, the discrepancy between costs, charges, and reimbursement, and the heterogeneous inclusion of direct and indirect cost between studies make cost comparisons difficult to interpret.[99]

Nevertheless, the personal and economic burden of suffering from bladder cancer is substantial and likely to worsen as the population ages. Although the new technologies evaluated in this review represent some potentially promising advances, further efforts to discover and evaluate novel diagnostic, therapeutic, and surgical techniques are essential to move the study of bladder cancer forward.

REFERENCES

1. Riley GF, Potosky AL, Lubitz JD, et al. Medicare payments from diagnosis to death for elderly cancer patients by stage at diagnosis. Med Care 1995; 33(8):828–41.

2. Botteman MF, Pashos CL, Redaelli A, et al. The health economics of bladder cancer: a comprehensive review of the published literature. Pharmacoeconomics 2003;21(18):1315–30.

3. Yeung C, Dinh T, Lee J. The health economics of bladder cancer: an updated review of the published literature. Pharmacoeconomics 2014;32(11): 1093–104.

4. American Urological Association: Guideline for the management of nonmuscle invasive bladder cancer (stages ta, T1, and tis): 2007 update. Updated 2007. Available at: www.auanet.org. Accessed September 25, 2014.

5. Clark PE, Agarwal N, Biagioli MC, et al. Bladder cancer. J Natl Compr Canc Netw 2013;11(4):446–75.

6. Babjuk M, Burger M, Zigeuner R, et al. EAU guidelines on non-muscle-invasive urothelial carcinoma of the bladder: update 2013. Eur Urol 2013;64(4):639–53.

7. Shabsigh A, Korets R, Vora KC, et al. Defining early morbidity of radical cystectomy for patients with bladder cancer using a standardized reporting methodology. Eur Urol 2009;55(1):164–74.

8. Svatek RS, Fisher MB, Matin SF, et al. Risk factor analysis in a contemporary cystectomy cohort using standardized reporting methodology and adverse event criteria. J Urol 2010;183(3):929–34.

9. Johnson DC, Nielsen ME, Matthews J, et al. Neoadjuvant chemotherapy for bladder cancer does not increase risk of perioperative morbidity. BJU Int 2014;114(2):221–8.

10. Hu M, Jacobs BL, Montgomery JS, et al. Sharpening the focus on causes and timing of readmission after radical cystectomy for bladder cancer. Cancer 2014;120(9):1409–16.

11. Avritscher EB, Cooksley CD, Grossman HB, et al. Clinical model of lifetime cost of treating bladder cancer and associated complications. Urology 2006;68(3):549–53.

12. Yabroff KR, Bradley CJ, Mariotto AB, et al. Estimates and projections of value of life lost from cancer deaths in the united states. J Natl Cancer Inst 2008;100(24):1755–62.

13. Gore JL, Gilbert SM. Improving bladder cancer patient care: a pharmacoeconomic perspective. Expert Rev Anticancer Ther 2013;13(6):661–8.

14. Sievert KD, Amend B, Nagele U, et al. Economic aspects of bladder cancer: what are the benefits and costs? World J Urol 2009;27(3):295–300.

15. Sylvester RJ, van der Meijden AP, Oosterlinck W, et al. Predicting recurrence and progression in individual patients with stage Ta T1 bladder cancer using EORTC risk tables: a combined analysis of 2596 patients from seven EORTC trials. Eur Urol 2006;49(3):466–75 [discussion: 475–7].

16. Divrik RT, Sahin AF, Yildirim U, et al. Impact of routine second transurethral resection on the long-term outcome of patients with newly diagnosed pT1 urothelial carcinoma with respect to recurrence, progression rate, and disease-specific survival: a prospective randomised clinical trial. Eur Urol 2010;58(2):185–90.

17. Karaolides T, Skolarikos A, Bourdoumis A, et al. Hexaminolevulinate-induced fluorescence versus white light during transurethral resection of noninvasive bladder tumor: does it reduce recurrences? Urology 2012;80(2):354–9.

18. Burger M, Grossman HB, Droller M, et al. Photodynamic diagnosis of non-muscle-invasive bladder

cancer with hexaminolevulinate cystoscopy: a meta-analysis of detection and recurrence based on raw data. Eur Urol 2013;64(5):846–54.

19. Witjes JA, Babjuk M, Gontero P, et al. Clinical and cost effectiveness of hexaminolevulinate-guided blue-light cystoscopy: evidence review and updated expert recommendations. Eur Urol 2014;66 [pii: S0302-2838(14)00611-3].

20. Oude Elferink P, Witjes JA. Blue-light cystoscopy in the evaluation of non-muscle-invasive bladder cancer. Ther Adv Urol 2014;6(1):25–33.

21. Stenzl A, Burger M, Fradet Y, et al. Hexaminolevulinate guided fluorescence cystoscopy reduces recurrence in patients with nonmuscle invasive bladder cancer. J Urol 2010;184(5):1907–13.

22. Burger M, Stief CG, Zaak D, et al. Hexaminolevulinate is equal to 5-aminolevulinic acid concerning residual tumor and recurrence rate following photodynamic diagnostic assisted transurethral resection of bladder tumors. Urology 2009;74(6): 1282–6.

23. Marti A, Jichlinski P, Lange N, et al. Comparison of aminolevulinic acid and hexylester aminolevulinate induced protoporphyrin IX distribution in human bladder cancer. J Urol 2003;170(2 Pt 1):428–32.

24. Yuan H, Qiu J, Liu L, et al. Therapeutic outcome of fluorescence cystoscopy guided transurethral resection in patients with non-muscle invasive bladder cancer: a meta-analysis of randomized controlled trials. PLoS One 2013;8(9):e74142.

25. Rink M, Babjuk M, Catto JW, et al. Hexyl aminolevulinate-guided fluorescence cystoscopy in the diagnosis and follow-up of patients with non-muscle-invasive bladder cancer: a critical review of the current literature. Eur Urol 2013;64(4):624–38.

26. Witjes JA, Gomella LG, Stenzl A, et al. Safety of hexaminolevulinate for blue light cystoscopy in bladder cancer. A combined analysis of the trials used for registration and postmarketing data. Urology 2014;84(1):122–6.

27. Cysview (hexaminolevulinate hydrochloride), for intravesical solution - highlights of prescribing information. Updated 2010. Available at: http://www.accessdata.fda.gov/drugsatfda_docs/label/2010/022555s000lbl.pdf. Accessed October 3, 2014.

28. Bunce C, Ayres BE, Griffiths TR, et al. The role of hexylaminolaevulinate in the diagnosis and follow-up of non-muscle-invasive bladder cancer. BJU Int 2010;105(Suppl 2):2–7.

29. Malmstrom PU, Grabe M, Haug ES, et al. Role of hexaminolevulinate-guided fluorescence cystoscopy in bladder cancer: critical analysis of the latest data and European guidance. Scand J Urol Nephrol 2012;46(2):108–16.

30. Daneshmand S, Schuckman AK, Bochner BH, et al. Hexaminolevulinate blue-light cystoscopy in non-muscle-invasive bladder cancer: review of the clinical evidence and consensus statement on appropriate use in the USA. Nat Rev Urol 2014;11(10):589–96.

31. Dindyal S, Nitkunan T, Bunce CJ. The economic benefit of photodynamic diagnosis in non-muscle invasive bladder cancer. Photodiagnosis Photodyn Ther 2008;5(2):153–8.

32. Burger M, Zaak D, Stief CG, et al. Photodynamic diagnostics and noninvasive bladder cancer: is it cost-effective in long-term application? A Germany-based cost analysis. Eur Urol 2007;52(1):142–7.

33. Otto W, Burger M, Fritsche HM, et al. Photodynamic diagnosis for superficial bladder cancer: do all risk-groups profit equally from oncological and economic long-term results? Clin Med Oncol 2009;3:53–8.

34. Malmstrom PU, Hedelin H, Thomas YK, et al. Fluorescence-guided transurethral resection of bladder cancer using hexaminolevulinate: analysis of health economic impact in Sweden. Scand J Urol Nephrol 2009;43(3):192–8.

35. Garfield SS, Gavaghan MB, Armstrong SO, et al. The cost-effectiveness of blue light cystoscopy in bladder cancer detection: United States projections based on clinical data showing 4.5 years of follow up after a single hexaminolevulinate hydrochloride instillation. Can J Urol 2013;20(2):6682–9.

36. Grossman HB, Stenzl A, Fradet Y, et al. Long-term decrease in bladder cancer recurrence with hexaminolevulinate enabled fluorescence cystoscopy. J Urol 2012;188(1):58–62.

37. Marteau F, Kornowski A, Bennison C, et al. Cost-effectiveness of the optical imaging agent hexaminolevulinate for patients undergoing initial transurethral resection of non-muscle invasive bladder cancer tumours. Eur Urol Suppl 2013;12(125) [abstract: 01].

38. O'Brien T, Ray E, Chatterton K, et al. Prospective randomized trial of hexylaminolevulinate photodynamic-assisted transurethral resection of bladder tumour (TURBT) plus single-shot intravesical mitomycin C vs conventional white-light TURBT plus mitomycin C in newly presenting non-muscle-invasive bladder cancer. BJU Int 2013;112(8):1096–104.

39. Geavlete B, Multescu R, Georgescu D, et al. Treatment changes and long-term recurrence rates after hexaminolevulinate (HAL) fluorescence cystoscopy: does it really make a difference in patients with non-muscle-invasive bladder cancer (NMIBC)? BJU Int 2012;109(4):549–56.

40. Menon M, Hemal AK, Tewari A, et al. Nerve-sparing robot-assisted radical cystoprostatectomy and urinary diversion. BJU Int 2003;92(3):232–6.

41. Leow JJ, Reese SW, Jiang W, et al. Propensity-matched comparison of morbidity and costs of open and robot-assisted radical cystectomies: a contemporary population-based analysis in the united states. Eur Urol 2014;66(3):569–76.

42. Monn MF, Cary KC, Kaimakliotis HZ, et al. National trends in the utilization of robotic-assisted radical

cystectomy: an analysis using the nationwide inpatient sample. Urol Oncol 2014;32(6):785–90.

43. Li K, Lin T, Fan X, et al. Systematic review and meta-analysis of comparative studies reporting early outcomes after robot-assisted radical cystectomy versus open radical cystectomy. Cancer Treat Rev 2013;39(6):551–60.

44. Tang K, Xia D, Li H, et al. Robotic vs open radical cystectomy in bladder cancer: a systematic review and meta-analysis. Eur J Surg Oncol 2014;40(11):1399–411.

45. Ishii H, Rai BP, Stolzenburg JU, et al. Robotic or open radical cystectomy, which is safer? A systematic review and meta-analysis of comparative studies. J Endourol 2014;28(10):1215–23.

46. Nix J, Smith A, Kurpad R, et al. Prospective randomized controlled trial of robotic versus open radical cystectomy for bladder cancer: perioperative and pathologic results. Eur Urol 2010;57(2):196–201.

47. Kader AK, Richards KA, Krane LS, et al. Robot-assisted laparoscopic vs open radical cystectomy: comparison of complications and perioperative oncological outcomes in 200 patients. BJU Int 2013;112(4):E290–4.

48. Niegisch G, Albers P, Rabenalt R. Perioperative complications and oncological safety of robot-assisted (RARC) vs open radical cystectomy (ORC). Urol Oncol 2014;32(7):966–74.

49. Musch M, Janowski M, Steves A, et al. Comparison of early postoperative morbidity after robot-assisted and open radical cystectomy: results of a prospective observational study. BJU Int 2014;113(3):458–67.

50. Ahdoot M, Almario L, Araya H, et al. Oncologic outcomes between open and robotic-assisted radical cystectomy: a propensity score matched analysis. World J Urol 2014;32(6):1441–6.

51. Merseburger AS, Herrmann TR, Shariat SF, et al. EAU guidelines on robotic and single-site surgery in urology. Eur Urol 2013;64(2):277–91.

52. Parekh DJ, Messer J, Fitzgerald J, et al. Perioperative outcomes and oncologic efficacy from a pilot prospective randomized clinical trial of open versus robotic assisted radical cystectomy. J Urol 2013;189(2):474–9.

53. Bochner BH, Sjoberg DD, Laudone VP, Memorial Sloan Kettering Cancer Center Bladder Cancer Surgical Trials Group. A randomized trial of robot-assisted laparoscopic radical cystectomy. N Engl J Med 2014;371(4):389–90.

54. Keren Paz GE, Laudone VP, Bochner BH. Does minimally invasive surgery for radical cystectomy provide similar long-term cancer control as open radical surgery? Curr Opin Urol 2013;23(5):449–55.

55. Khan MS, Elhage O, Challacombe B, et al. Long-term outcomes of robot-assisted radical cystectomy for bladder cancer. Eur Urol 2013;64(2):219–24.

56. Snow-Lisy DC, Campbell SC, Gill IS, et al. Robotic and laparoscopic radical cystectomy for bladder cancer: long-term oncologic outcomes. Eur Urol 2014;65(1):193–200.

57. Smith A, Kurpad R, Lal A, et al. Cost analysis of robotic versus open radical cystectomy for bladder cancer. J Urol 2010;183(2):505–9.

58. Martin AD, Nunez RN, Castle EP. Robot-assisted radical cystectomy versus open radical cystectomy: a complete cost analysis. Urology 2011;77(3):621–5.

59. Lee R, Chughtai B, Herman M, et al. Cost-analysis comparison of robot-assisted laparoscopic radical cystectomy (RC) vs open RC. BJU Int 2011;108(6 Pt 2):976–83.

60. Ahmed K, Khan MS, Vats A, et al. Current status of robotic assisted pelvic surgery and future developments. Int J Surg 2009;7(5):431–40.

61. Yu HY, Hevelone ND, Lipsitz SR, et al. Comparative analysis of outcomes and costs following open radical cystectomy versus robot-assisted laparoscopic radical cystectomy: results from the US nationwide inpatient sample. Eur Urol 2012;61(6):1239–44.

62. Hardt J, Filipas D, Hohenfellner R, et al. Quality of life in patients with bladder carcinoma after cystectomy: first results of a prospective study. Qual Life Res 2000;9(1):1–12.

63. Kulaksizoglu H, Toktas G, Kulaksizoglu IB, et al. When should quality of life be measured after radical cystectomy? Eur Urol 2002;42(4):350–5.

64. Stegemann A, Rehman S, Brewer K, et al. Short-term patient-reported quality of life after robot-assisted radical cystectomy using the convalescence and recovery evaluation. Urology 2012;79(6):1274–9.

65. Poch MA, Stegemann AP, Rehman S, et al. Short-term patient reported health-related quality of life (HRQL) outcomes after robot-assisted radical cystectomy (RARC). BJU Int 2014;113(2):260–5.

66. Messer JC, Punnen S, Fitzgerald J, et al. Health-related quality of life from a prospective randomised clinical trial of robot-assisted laparoscopic vs open radical cystectomy. BJU Int 2014;114(6):896–902.

67. Aboumohamed AA, Raza SJ, Al-Daghmin A, et al. Health-related quality of life outcomes after robot-assisted and open radical cystectomy using a validated bladder-specific instrument: a multi-institutional study. Urology 2014;83(6):1300–8.

68. Smith ND, Castle EP, Gonzalgo ML, et al. The RAZOR trial (randomized open versus robotic cystectomy): study design and trial update. BJU Int 2015;115(2):198–205.

69. Chang SS, Cookson MS, Baumgartner RG, et al. Analysis of early complications after radical cystectomy: results of a collaborative care pathway. J Urol 2002;167(5):2012–6.

70. Cookson MS, Chang SS, Wells N, et al. Complications of radical cystectomy for nonmuscle invasive

disease: comparison with muscle invasive disease. J Urol 2003;169(1):101–4.

71. Hollenbeck BK, Miller DC, Taub D, et al. Identifying risk factors for potentially avoidable complications following radical cystectomy. J Urol 2005;174(4 Pt 1):1231–7 [discussion: 1237].

72. Donat SM, Shabsigh A, Savage C, et al. Potential impact of postoperative early complications on the timing of adjuvant chemotherapy in patients undergoing radical cystectomy: a high-volume tertiary cancer center experience. Eur Urol 2009;55(1): 177–85.

73. Svatek RS, Fisher MB, Williams MB, et al. Age and body mass index are independent risk factors for the development of postoperative paralytic ileus after radical cystectomy. Urology 2010;76(6):1419–24.

74. Liu SS, Hodgson PS, Carpenter RL, et al. ADL 8-2698, a trans-3,4-dimethyl-4-(3-hydroxyphenyl) piperidine, prevents gastrointestinal effects of intravenous morphine without affecting analgesia. Clin Pharmacol Ther 2001;69(1):66–71.

75. Entereg (alvimopan) prescribing information. Available at: http://www.entereg.com/content/pdf/entereg_prescribing_information.pdf. Accessed October 20, 2014.

76. McNicol ED, Boyce D, Schumann R, et al. Mu-opioid antagonists for opioid-induced bowel dysfunction. Cochrane Database Syst Rev 2008;(2):CD006332.

77. Wolff BG, Michelassi F, Gerkin TM, et al. Alvimopan, a novel, peripherally acting mu opioid antagonist: results of a multicenter, randomized, double-blind, placebo-controlled, phase III trial of major abdominal surgery and postoperative ileus. Ann Surg 2004;240(4):728–34 [discussion: 734–5].

78. Delaney CP, Weese JL, Hyman NH, et al. Phase III trial of alvimopan, a novel, peripherally acting, mu opioid antagonist, for postoperative ileus after major abdominal surgery. Dis Colon Rectum 2005;48(6): 1114–25.

79. Viscusi ER, Goldstein S, Witkowski T, et al. Alvimopan, a peripherally acting mu-opioid receptor antagonist, compared with placebo in postoperative ileus after major abdominal surgery: results of a randomized, double-blind, controlled study. Surg Endosc 2006;20(1):64–70.

80. Ludwig K, Enker WE, Delaney CP, et al. Gastrointestinal tract recovery in patients undergoing bowel resection: results of a randomized trial of alvimopan and placebo with a standardized accelerated postoperative care pathway. Arch Surg 2008;143(11): 1098–105.

81. Buchler MW, Seiler CM, Monson JR, et al. Clinical trial: alvimopan for the management of postoperative ileus after abdominal surgery: results of an international randomized, double-blind, multicentre, placebo-controlled clinical study. Aliment Pharmacol Ther 2008;28(3):312–25.

82. Cerantola Y, Valerio M, Persson B, et al. Guidelines for perioperative care after radical cystectomy for bladder cancer: enhanced recovery after surgery (ERAS((R))) society recommendations. Clin Nutr 2013;32(6):879–87.

83. Karl A, Buchner A, Becker A, et al. A new concept for early recovery after surgery for patients undergoing radical cystectomy for bladder cancer: results of a prospective randomized study. J Urol 2014;191(2): 335–40.

84. Smith J, Meng ZW, Lockyer R, et al. Evolution of the Southampton enhanced recovery programme for radical cystectomy and the aggregation of marginal gains. BJU Int 2014;114(3):375–83.

85. Dutton TJ, Daugherty MO, Mason RG, et al. Implementation of the Exeter enhanced recovery programme for patients undergoing radical cystectomy. BJU Int 2014;113(5):719–25.

86. Vora A, Marchalik D, Nissim H, et al. Multi-institutional outcomes and cost effectiveness of using alvimopan to lower gastrointestinal morbidity after cystectomy and urinary diversion. Can J Urol 2014; 21(2):7222–7.

87. Lee CT, Chang SS, Kamat AM, et al. Alvimopan accelerates gastrointestinal recovery after radical cystectomy: a multicenter randomized placebo-controlled trial. Eur Urol 2014;66(2):265–72.

88. Kraft M, Maclaren R, Du W, et al. Alvimopan (entereg) for the management of postoperative ileus in patients undergoing bowel resection. P T 2010; 35(1):44–9.

89. Bell TJ, Poston SA, Kraft MD, et al. Economic analysis of alvimopan in north american phase III efficacy trials. Am J Health Syst Pharm 2009;66(15): 1362–8.

90. Poston S, Broder MS, Gibbons MM, et al. Impact of alvimopan (entereg) on hospital costs after bowel resection: results from a large inpatient database. P T 2011;36(4):209–20.

91. Delaney CP, Craver C, Gibbons MM, et al. Evaluation of clinical outcomes with alvimopan in clinical practice: a national matched-cohort study in patients undergoing bowel resection. Ann Surg 2012; 255(4):731–8.

92. Touchette DR, Yang Y, Tiryaki F, et al. Economic analysis of alvimopan for prevention and management of postoperative ileus. Pharmacotherapy 2012;32(2):120–8.

93. Hilton WM, Lotan Y, Parekh DJ, et al. Alvimopan for prevention of postoperative paralytic ileus in radical cystectomy patients: a cost-effectiveness analysis. BJU Int 2013;111(7):1054–60.

94. Kauf TL, Svatek RS, Amiel G, et al. Alvimopan, a peripherally acting mu-opioid receptor antagonist, is associated with reduced costs after radical cystectomy: economic analysis of a phase 4 randomized, controlled trial. J Urol 2014;191(6):1721–7.

95. Siegel R, Ma J, Zou Z, et al. Cancer statistics, 2014. CA Cancer J Clin 2014;64(1):9–29.

96. Lotan Y, Kamat AM, Porter MP, et al. Key concerns about the current state of bladder cancer: a position paper from the bladder cancer think tank, the bladder cancer advocacy network, and the society of urologic oncology. Cancer 2009;115(18):4096–103.

97. Carter AJ, Nguyen CN. A comparison of cancer burden and research spending reveals discrepancies in the distribution of research funding. BMC Public Health 2012;12:526.

98. Noyes K, Singer EA, Messing EM. Healthcare economics of bladder cancer: cost-enhancing and cost-reducing factors. Curr Opin Urol 2008;18(5):533–9.

99. Zehnder P, Gill IS. Cost-effectiveness of open versus laparoscopic versus robotic-assisted laparoscopic cystectomy and urinary diversion. Curr Opin Urol 2011;21(5):415–9.

Targeted Therapy in Advanced Bladder Cancer
What Have We Learned?

Emmet J. Jordan, MB BCh, BAO, MRCPI, Gopa Iyer, MD*

KEYWORDS

- Urothelial carcinoma • Targeted therapy • Small molecule inhibitors • Next-generation sequencing
- Angiogenesis • MAPK pathway • PI3K/Akt/mTOR pathway

KEY POINTS

- Clinical trials of targeted agents in urothelial carcinoma have not displayed a significant improvement in response or outcome compared with chemotherapy.
- None of these trials have incorporated prospective sequencing to identify predictive biomarkers of response to therapy.
- Predictive biomarkers are crucial for identifying patients most likely to obtain benefit from targeted agents.
- Basket clinical studies will allow targeted agents to be assessed across tumor types based on the presence of a specific genetic biomarker.

BACKGROUND

Urothelial carcinoma (UC) is the second most common genitourinary malignancy in the United States, with an estimated 74,690 new cases and 15,580 estimated deaths in 2014.[1] For locally advanced or metastatic UC, first-line cisplatin-based chemotherapy results in an overall response rate (ORR) of 50% to 70%, a median progression-free survival (PFS) of 7 to 9 months, and median overall survival (OS) of 12 to 15 months.[2] The doublet of gemcitabine plus cisplatin (GC) offers similar survival rates to that of the 4-drug regimen of methotrexate, vinblastine, doxorubicin, and cisplatin with a median survival of 14.0 months (95% confidence interval [CI], 12.3–15.5 months) versus 15.2 months (95% CI, 13.2–17.3 months), respectively. Although these survival outcomes outstrip the estimated 6-month survival rates observed before these regimens, advances are indisputably needed.[2] The addition of paclitaxel to GC chemotherapy improved response rates but did not show a significant improvement in median survival and resulted in increased toxicity,[3] whereas the use of dose-dense therapies have to date not resulted in improvements in OS.[4] These results, coupled with the success of targeted agents in other cancer types such as renal cell carcinoma (RCC), non–small cell lung cancer (NSCLC), and chronic myelogenous leukemia, have driven the search to define a role for targeted therapies in advanced UC.

GENETIC ALTERATIONS IN UROTHELIAL CARCINOMA

Sequencing of UC tumors initially identified 2 distinct mutation patterns, which correlated with tumor grade. Low-grade papillary tumors were characterized primarily by oncogenic mutations in the fibroblast growth factor receptor 3 (FGFR3; ~70%), HRAS (30%–40%), and PIK3CA (~10%)

Disclosure Statement: The authors indicate no conflicts of interest.
Department of Medicine, Memorial Sloan Kettering Cancer Center, 1275 York Avenue, New York, NY 10065, USA
* Corresponding author.
E-mail address: iyerg@mskcc.org

Urol Clin N Am 42 (2015) 253–262
http://dx.doi.org/10.1016/j.ucl.2015.01.006

genes.[5] Conversely, invasive lesions harbored frequent loss of function alterations in tumor suppressor genes, including *TP53* and *RB1*.[6,7] The Cancer Genome Atlas (TCGA) has since provided a more granular insight into the landscape of genetic alterations within muscle-invasive UC.[8] Despite a high mutation burden, many alterations can be organized into well-known signaling pathways and canonical cellular functions against which inhibitors have been approved by the US Food and Drug Administration (FDA) in other cancer types or are currently under investigation.[9] These pathways primarily include the receptor tyrosine kinase (RTK) pathway, comprised of the epidermal growth factor receptor (EGFR) family of receptors, FGFR3, and numerous others, and the phosphoinositide 3-kinase (PI3K)/Akt/ mammalian target of rapamycin (mTOR) pathway. Additionally, UC is characterized by a high frequency of alterations within cell cycle regulatory genes, including *CDKN2A* deletion and *CCND1* amplification. Chromatin modifiers such as *KDM6A*, *KMT2D*, and *ARID1A* represent another class of genes commonly mutated in this disease. Finally, angiogenesis is thought to play a key role in UC growth and metastatic spread, and components of this signaling axis are also altered in UC. Most targeted therapy trials performed thus far in UC have investigated RTK and angiogenic signaling inhibitors and mTOR inhibitors. These studies are the focus of this discussion and are outlined in **Table 1**.

RECEPTOR TYROSINE KINASE SIGNALING INHIBITORS
Epidermal Growth Factor Receptor Signaling

EGFR (Erbb1) is a 170-kDa transmembrane RTK critically important for the regulation of cell proliferation, invasion, and metastasis in preclinical models of UC.[10] Activation of the EGFR-tyrosine kinase (TK) stimulates both the MAPK and PI3K/ Akt/mTOR signaling pathways. Additional members of the ErbB family of receptors also involved in mitogenic signaling via the MAPK pathway include HER2 and HER3. EGFR and HER2 have both been examined as potential targets in UC. In the bladder TCGA, comprised of untreated muscle-invasive specimens, MAPK pathway alterations include EGFR amplification (9%), HER2 amplifications and mutations (9%), and HER3 mutations (6%).

Gefitinib
Gefitinib is an oral, selective EGFR TK inhibitor currently used in EGFR-mutant NSCLC patients and has activity against EGFR-expressing UC

cell lines.[11] Gefitinib was evaluated in a phase II trial in metastatic UC patients who did not respond to one prior chemotherapeutic regimen. In the 31 patients enrolled, the median PFS was 2 months with one confirmed partial response (PR).[12] Pretreatment biopsies were required for retrospective evaluation of EGFR expression, although overexpression was not an inclusion criterion. The partial responder's tumor harbored 2+ EGFR expression; 8 of 15 patients showed primary progression (2 to 3+ EGFR expression). No correlation was noted between EGFR staining and response; additionally, this study was designed before the observation that EGFR mutations correlate with gefitinib sensitivity in NSCLC.

The Cancer and Leukemia Group B conducted a multicenter phase II study (CALGB 90102) evaluating the addition of gefitinib (500 mg/d) to GC in untreated patients with advanced UC.[13] All patients received 6 cycles of GC plus gefitinib, and those with objective responses or stable disease (SD) were continued on maintenance gefitinib until progression. An ORR of 42.6% was observed with 7 complete responses (CR) and 16 PRs. The median OS was 15.1 months; the median time to progression was 7.4 months. Grades 3 to 4 hematologic toxicity were seen in 22% patients (n = 12). Nonhematologic grade 3 toxicities included fatigue (20%), emesis (24%), diarrhea (14%), and rash (11%). Based on these results, the addition of gefitinib does not seem to improve response rate or survival compared with chemotherapy alone. Notably, patients were not screened for EGFR overexpression or mutation before trial enrollment.

Erlotinib
Erlotinib, another EGFR TK inhibitor, was tested in 20 patients with histologically confirmed muscle-invasive UC in the neoadjuvant setting for 4 weeks before radical cystectomy.[14] Seven patients (35%) with clinical T2 disease had their disease downstaged to non-muscle-invasive bladder cancer, and 5 patients (25%) had no residual disease, comparing favorably with historical rates of less than pT2 disease after transurethral resection or neoadjuvant chemotherapy, although the lack of a comparator arm in this study limits the ability to draw definitive conclusions. Treatment was well tolerated with rash the most common side effect observed in 15 patients (75%). Five patients who achieved pT0 responses within the bladder exhibited the acneiform rash known to correlate with response to EGFR TK inhibition in NSCLC and colon cancers. Although patients were not preselected based on EGFR mutations or amplification, tumors are being retrospectively analyzed

Table 1
Clinical trials of targeted agents in urothelial carcinoma

Targeted Therapy	No. of Patients		Response Rate	Median PFS (mo)	Median OS (mo)
EGFR					
Gefitinib[12]	31	Second line	3%	2	3
Gefitinib[13]	58	First line +GC	42.6%	7.4	15.1
Erlotinib[14]	20	Neoadjuvant	60%	N/A	N/A
Cetuximab[19]	28	Second line ± paclitaxel	25%	16.4 wk	42 wk
Cetuximab[20]	88	First line +GC	57.1% (GC) vs 61.4% (GC+ Ctx)	8.5 (GC) vs 7.6 (GC + Ctx)	17.4 (GC) vs 14.3 (GC + Ctx)
EGFR + Her2					
Lapatinib[15]	59	Second line	1.7%	8.6 wk	17.9 wk
Her2					
Trastuzumab[24]	44	First line + PCaG	70%	9.3	14.1
FGFR3					
Dovitinib[28]	44	Second line, FGFR3 wt and mut	3% (wt) 0% (mut)	1.8 (wt) 3 (mut)	NR
Angiogenesis					
Sunitinib[38]	77	Second line			
		50 mg daily 4 wk on/2 wk off	7%	2.4	7.1
		37.5 mg daily	3%	2.3	6
Sunitinib[40]	38	First-line cisplatin ineligible	8%	4.8	8.1
Sorafenib[41]	17	First line	0%	1.9	5.9
Sorafenib[42]	22	Second line	0%	2.2	6.8
Sorafenib[43]	40	First line ± GC	52.5%	6.3	11.3
Pazopanib[45]	41	Second line	17.1%	2.6	4.7
Bevacizumab[54]	43	First line + GC	72%	8.2	19.1
Bevacizumab[55]	51	First line + GCa	49%	6.5	13.9
mTOR					
Everolimus[61]	37	Second line	27%	61 d	101 d
Everolimus[62]	45	Second line	5%**	2.6	8.3
VEGFR + EGFR					
Vandetanib[46]	142	Second line ± docetaxel	7%	2.56	5.85

**, proportion of patients exhibiting a CR plus PR.
Abbreviations: Ctx, Cetuximab; GCa, Gemcitabine + Carboplatin; mut, mutant; N/A, Not applicable; NR, Not reported; PCaG, Paclitaxel + Carboplatin + Gemcitabine; wt, wild-type.
Data from Refs.[12–15,19,20,24,28,38,40–43,45,46,54,55,61,62]

to define any molecular correlates with treatment response.

Lapatinib
Lapatinib, a dual TK inhibitor of EGFR and HER2, was evaluated as second-line therapy in 59 platinum-refractory locally advanced or metastatic UC patients with a primary endpoint of objective response rate greater than 10%.[15] One patient achieved a PR; 18 (31%) patients displayed SD.

Median time to disease progression and OS were 8.6 weeks and 17.9 weeks, respectively. Diarrhea, nausea, and vomiting were the most commonly reported toxicities. Seventeen of 19 patients who achieved SD or PR (89%) had EGFR and/or HER2 overexpressing tumors. The possible correlation between EGFR and HER2 expression and response to lapatinib therapy underscores the importance of prospective genetic sequencing as an eligibility criterion for targeted therapy studies.

Cetuximab

Cetuximab is an anti-EGFR monoclonal antibody FDA approved for the treatment of head and neck and colorectal cancers.[16–18] A randomized phase II study gauged the efficacy of cetuximab with or without paclitaxel in patients with previously treated metastatic UC.[19] Patients received weekly cetuximab alone or weekly paclitaxel plus cetuximab. The single-agent cetuximab arm was terminated after 9 of the first 11 patients exhibited progression at 8 weeks. Median PFS and OS were 7.6 weeks and 17 weeks, respectively, and no objective responses were observed. In contrast, 28 patients were enrolled onto the combination arm with a median PFS and OS of 16.4 weeks and 42 weeks, respectively. The ORR was 25% (3 CRs and 4 PRs). Notably, the most common treatment-related grade 3 to 4 adverse events were rash and hypomagnesemia. A comparator arm using single-agent chemotherapy was not incorporated into this study. Additionally, patients who received perioperative chemotherapy but not first-line therapy in the metastatic setting were also enrolled. Finally, patients were not preselected based on molecular predictors of response or resistance to cetuximab, such as EGFR overexpression or KRAS mutation, respectively.

A randomized phase II trial of GC with or without cetuximab was performed in advanced UC patients, with a primary endpoint of ORR. Patients were randomly assigned in a 1:2 fashion to GC alone or GC with cetuximab.[20] Early in the study, gemcitabine was dose reduced by 20% to mitigate an observed increase in thromboembolic events with the 3-drug combination, resulting in decreased standard-of-care dose intensity. The ORR was 57.1% with GC and 61.4% with GC plus cetuximab. The median OS was 17.4 months with GC versus 14.3 months with GC plus cetuximab ($P = .43$). A higher rate of grades 3 to 4 acneiform rash was seen with cetuximab.

Trastuzumab

HER2 overexpression has been linked to shorter time to recurrence and is found in both primary and metastatic lesions in UC.[21,22] Micropapillary histology, an aggressive variant characterized by poor survival, also harbors a high rate of *ERBB2* amplification.[23] In a retrospective analysis of 80 UC specimens derived from radical cystectomies, 28% exhibited 2 to 3+ HER2 overexpression by immunohistochemistry (IHC). In 60 of these specimens, matched metastatic samples were available, and 2 to 3+ HER2 overexpression was observed in both lymph node (63%) and distant (86%) metastatic deposits. Based on these findings, a trial assessing the safety and efficacy of the humanized monoclonal anti-HER2 antibody, trastuzumab, in combination with carboplatin, gemcitabine, and paclitaxel in advanced UC patients was conducted, with cardiac toxicity as the primary endpoint.[24] HER2 overexpression by IHC, gene amplification by fluorescence in situ hybridization (FISH), or elevated serum extracellular domain HER2 levels was a requirement for study participation. The median time to progression and OS were 9.3 and 14.1 months, respectively, and the ORR was 70%, with most responses occurring in HER2 IHC 3+ or FISH-amplified patients. Because this was not a randomized trial, the impact of trastuzumab addition to chemotherapy could not be assessed. Additionally, the concordance between IHC overexpression and FISH amplification seen in breast cancer was not observed in this sample set, suggesting that gene amplification does not necessarily correlate with HER2 protein levels in UC.

Although the bladder TCGA identified HER2 alterations in 9% of muscle-invasive specimens, the HER2 mutation rate was higher than that of any other cancer type sequenced. Stemming from these data, neratinib, an irreversible HER2 TK inhibitor, which has shown significant improvements in disease-free survival in HER2+ breast cancer, is currently being tested in UC through a novel basket trial design.[25,26] Patients with EGFR mutations or amplifications and HER2 or HER3 mutations across multiple cancer types, including advanced UC, are being enrolled, with the primary objective of measuring 8-week ORR.

Fibroblast Growth Factor Receptor 3 Signaling

Fibroblast growth factors (FGFs) are involved in a variety of cellular processes, such as proliferation, antiapoptosis, and angiogenesis. FGFR3 is a particularly promising target for therapy in UC with an alteration rate of 16% in the bladder TCGA, including mutations (11%), amplifications (3%), and fusions (2%). Dovitinib, BGJ398, Ki23057, ponatinib, and AZD4547 are orally bioavailable FGFR inhibitors that have demonstrated efficacy in preclinical models of UC.[27]

Dovitinib

Dovitinib (TKI258), an oral multitargeted receptor TK inhibitor of FGFR1-3, vascular endothelial growth factor receptor (VEGFR), and others was assessed in 44 patients with metastatic chemo-refractory UC at a dose of 500 mg/d on a 5-days-on/2-days-off schedule.[28] The study included FGFR3 mutant and wild-type cases. None of the FGFR3 mutant patients responded; 1 PR was present in the wild-type cohort. The median PFS was 3 months in the mutant group and 1.8 months in the wild-type group. The drug was not carried into an expansion phase based on these results. A phase I study of BGJ398, a pan-FGFR inhibitor, in patients with metastatic FGFR-altered cancers, has shown promising results: 4 of 5 patients with FGFR3-mutant UC experienced tumor reductions (27%–48%), with hyperphosphatemia the most common adverse event noted.[29]

Tumor Angiogenesis

VEGF is one of the key angiogenic factors that stimulate the formation of new blood vessels.[30] Heightened levels of VEGF and interleukin (IL)-8 correlate with higher stage and a worse disease-free survival in advanced UC.[31–34] Microvessel density, a surrogate for tumor angiogenesis, was linked to disease recurrence when measured in UC biopsy specimens, and microvessel density was an independent prognostic factor associated with both disease-free survival and OS in a multivariate analysis of 164 invasive UC specimens.[35,36] These observations highlight the potential role for antiangiogenic agents in UC, and the success of these compounds in other malignancies has driven further investigation in this disease.

Sunitinib

Sunitinib is a small-molecule multitargeted receptor TK inhibitor against VEGFR, platelet-derived growth factor receptor, and KIT, with activity in in vitro and in vivo UC models.[37] In 77 patients with advanced, previously treated UC, sunitinib was assessed in 2 patient cohorts by dose and schedule: cohort A patients received 50 mg daily on a 4-week-on and 2-week-off regimen, whereas cohort B patients received 37.5 mg daily continuously.[38] Three patients in cohort A and 1 in cohort B experienced a PR. Clinical regression or stable disease was observed in 33 of 77 patients (43%); the duration of regression ranged from 0.6 to 23.4 months. PFS (2.4 vs 2.3 months) and OS (7.1 vs 6.0 months) were comparable between cohorts A and B, respectively. Grades 3 to 4 toxicities were observed in 57 patients. Sunitinib did not achieve the threshold of $\geq$20% ORR (CR + PR) to be considered promising; however, antitumor responses were seen in some patients, indicating that anti-VEGF signaling may be therapeutically effective in a biomarker-guided context. Additionally, tumor necrosis resulted in decreased density of marker lesions but did not correlate with reduction in tumor diameter, implying that the Response Evaluation Criteria in Solid Tumors (RECIST) may not be the most accurate method to gauge responses to anti-angiogenic agents. In the metastatic and neoadjuvant (muscle invasive disease) settings, the combination of gemcitabine and

cisplatin was assessed with sunitinib in 2 parallel phase II trials.[39] Both studies were limited by severe toxicity requiring premature closure.

Another multicenter trial evaluated sunitinib as first-line treatment in cisplatin-ineligible metastatic UC patients.[40] Of 38 patients, 3 (8%) evinced PRs and 19 (50%) exhibited stable disease. The median time to progression and OS were 4.8 months and 8.1 months, respectively, lower than the historical response rates observed with carboplatin-based chemotherapy. However, the 58% clinical benefit rate (PR+CR+SD) suggests activity in select patients. Notably, low pretreatment IL-8 levels correlated with improved time to progression. Additionally, patients with greater than 40 Hounsfield Unit enhancement within their tumors, a surrogate for high tumor vascularity on baseline contrast-enhanced computed tomography scans, were likelier to benefit from sunitinib.

Sorafenib

Sorafenib, another oral multitargeted receptor TK inhibitor against Raf and VEGFRs has also been evaluated in UC in 2 phase II trials: one in treatment-naïve metastatic disease and another in chemo-refractory patients. Neither study found any objective responses.[41,42] A randomized phase II trial in the first-line metastatic setting combined sorafenib or placebo with GC.[43] There were no significant differences in ORR or median PFS or OS between the 2 arms; diarrhea and hand-foot syndrome were more common with sorafenib therapy.

Pazopanib

Pazopanib is an oral multitargeted receptor TK inhibitor against VEGFR-1, -2, and -3; platelet-derived growth factor receptor–α and –β; and KIT.[44] This drug was FDA approved for first-line treatment of clear cell RCC. A phase II study assessed the efficacy of pazopanib, 800 mg daily, in patients with chemorefractory UC.[45] Twenty-one (51%) of 41 patients received pazopanib as third-line or further treatment, and 24% had an Eastern Cooperative Oncology Group (ECOG) performance status of 2. Seven patients had a confirmed PR (17.1%). The median PFS and OS were 2.6 and 4.7 months, respectively. Grade 3 toxicities were observed in 12 (29%) patients, including 2 cases each of gastrointestinal and vaginal fistulization; all 4 patients reinitiated therapy. One additional patient died of a duodenal fistula.[45] Patients who had fistulas also had bulky disease that responded significantly. On multivariate analysis, the presence of liver metastases, upper tract primary disease, and ECOG performance status were significantly associated with OS. When measured 4 weeks after treatment, IL-8 levels $\geq$87 pg/mL correlated with inferior OS (4.2 months vs 6.7 months for patients whose 4-week IL-8 levels were <87 pg/mL). The study investigators postulated that elevations in IL-8 levels within 4 weeks of treatment may reflect a resistance mechanism to anti-angiogenic therapy, thereby serving as an early predictive marker of lack of efficacy.

Vandetanib

Vandetanib, a dual VEGFR and EGFR inhibitor, was assessed in a randomized, phase II study with docetaxel in patients with advanced UC whose disease had progressed on platinum-based chemotherapy.[46] One hundred forty-two patients were randomly assigned to vandetanib, 100 mg daily plus docetaxel, or docetaxel plus placebo. The primary endpoint of this study was to compare PFS between the 2 arms. The median PFS was 2.56 months for docetaxel plus vandetanib versus 1.58 months for docetaxel plus placebo with an HR of 1.02 (95% CI, 0.69 to 1.49; $P = .9$). Response rates and OS were not different between the arms with a higher rate of toxicity in the combination arm including rash/photosensitivity (11% vs 0%) and diarrhea (7% vs 0%). When a validated prognostic model in patients whose disease progressed on platinum-based chemotherapy comprising Hgb less than 10 g/dL, ECOG PS greater than 0, and the presence of liver metastases was applied to the study population, all 3 parameters were significantly associated with a risk of death.[47]

Bevacizumab

Bevacizumab is a recombinant humanized monoclonal antibody against circulating VEGF and has displayed improvements in clinical outcomes when combined with chemotherapy in advanced RCC, NSCLC, colorectal cancer, and glioblastoma multiforme.[48–53] The Hoosier Oncology Group designed a phase II trial of GC plus bevacizumab (dosed at 15 mg/kg every 3 weeks) in chemotherapy-naive patients with metastatic or unresectable UC.[54] After 8 cycles of combination therapy, bevacizumab was continued for a total of 12 months. Because of a higher-than-expected thromboembolic rate, the gemcitabine dose was reduced from 1250 to 1000 mg/m². Deep vein thrombosis and pulmonary embolism events were subsequently significantly lower (8% after vs 41% before dose reduction; $P = .023$). Grades 3 to 4 hematologic toxicities included neutropenia, anemia, and thrombocytopenia. Nonhematologic grades 3 to 5 toxicities included hypertension (5%), proteinuria (2%), hemorrhage (7%), and cardiac toxicity (7%). Eight patients (19%) experienced a CR and 23 patients (53%)

a PR. The median PFS and OS were 8.2 months and 19.1 months, respectively.

Bevacizumab was also evaluated in cisplatin-ineligible patients in a phase II study of gemcitabine, carboplatin, and bevacizumab, 15 mg/kg every 3 weeks.[55] Patients received an initial dose of bevacizumab, 10 mg/kg, 2 weeks before the first dose of chemotherapy to enhance tumor penetration by cytotoxic agents. After a maximum of 6 cycles of chemotherapy, bevacizumab was continued for a total of 18 cycles as tolerated. The dose of carboplatin was reduced from an area under the curve of 5 to 4.5 after 13 patients were enrolled because of excess hematologic toxicities at the higher dose. An objective response was seen in 23 (49%) patients (3 complete; 20 partial), and 11 (23%) had SD. The median PFS was 6.5 months. The most common grade 3 to 4 toxicity was neutropenia (31%), whereas thromboembolic events were the most common nonhematologic grade 3 to 4 toxicities (20%). The median OS was 13.9 months, superior to that of other studies of patients treated with carboplatin plus gemcitabine alone. Additionally, 28 patients continued on maintenance bevacizumab after completing 6 cycles of chemotherapy, and 9 displayed shrinkage of target sites on monotherapy, suggesting that VEGF axis inhibition alone is effective in select patients.

Given these promising results, a phase III randomized trial (CALGB 90601) of GC with or without bevacizumab in the first-line metastatic setting is ongoing.

PHOSPHOINOSITIDE 3-KINASE/AKT/ MAMMALIAN TARGET OF RAPAMYCIN SIGNALING

PI3K signaling results in activation of Akt, a central nexus within the cell that promotes growth and proliferation and inhibits apoptosis; *PIK3CA* activating mutations, *TSC1/2* mutations or deletions, and *AKT3* overexpression were detected in 42% of bladder TCGA samples. Akt upregulates mTOR, a serine-threonine kinase that forms 2 multiprotein complexes (mTORC1 and mTORC2), which regulate cell growth, motility, and proliferation.[56] In addition to Akt, mTOR activity is controlled by amino acid supply, hypoxia, and DNA damage; the mTOR inhibitor everolimus has been FDA approved in numerous cancer types, including RCC, pancreatic neuroendocrine tumors, and HER2-negative, hormone receptor–positive breast cancer.[57–59]

Everolimus

Initial in vitro studies found that mTOR blockade by everolimus inhibited proliferation, stimulated cell cycle arrest, and downregulated phosphorylated S6, a key effector of mTOR activity, within UC cell lines; these results were recapitulated in xenograft models. Based on these preclinical findings, everolimus was explored further as a potential therapeutic agent in UC.[60]

A multicenter phase II study assessed everolimus, 10 mg daily, in patients with advanced UC after prior platinum-based therapy.[61] The primary endpoint was a 2-month disease control rate, defined as CR, PR, or SD. Of 37 evaluable patients, 2 patients experienced a PR and 8 patients SD, with a disease control rate of 27% at 8 weeks. The median PFS and OS were 61 days and 101 days, respectively.[61] Fatigue (27%) and thrombocytopenia (13%) were the most frequent grade 3 to 4 toxicities observed. Potential biomarkers of response to everolimus were examined, including plasma levels of angiopoietin-1, endoglin, and PDGF-AB (all angiogenesis-regulating proteins). A statistically significant reduction in the level of these proteins was seen in patients with disease control as opposed to those with progressive disease. Loss of PTEN expression was observed in 57% of patients with progressive disease and in none of the patients who achieved disease control.

Another phase II study examined everolimus in 45 patients with advanced UC who had progressed on 1 to 4 prior lines of cytotoxic chemotherapy.[62] A median PFS of 2.6 (1.8–3.5) months and a median OS of 8.3 (5.5–12.1) months were observed. In 8 patients, treatment was stopped secondary to drug-related toxicities; common grade 3 to 4 toxicities included hyperglycemia, hypophosphatemia, and fatigue. Six patients experienced everolimus-related pneumonitis. Notably, one patient experienced a durable CR to treatment lasting greater than 26 months (ongoing). Whole genome sequencing of this patient's cystectomy specimen found alterations in TSC1 and NF2, which were predicted to result in premature truncation of both proteins. TSC1 and NF2 are negative regulators of the mTOR pathway, and inactivation of both proteins leads to enhanced mTOR signaling, suggesting that loss of both tumor suppressor proteins may have resulted in the depth and duration of response observed within this patient.[63] Exon capture sequencing of 13 additional patients on the study found 4 TSC1 alterations, 3 of which were present in patients with minor responses to therapy. This discovery reinforces the importance of the PI3K/AKT/mTOR signaling pathway as a potential target in UC and underscores the utility of prospective genotyping to identify those patients with pathway-altered tumors most likely to respond to mTOR-directed therapies.

ADDITIONAL TARGETS IN UROTHELIAL CARCINOMA

As mentioned before, cell cycle regulatory genes are frequently altered in UC, including CDKN2A (47% deletion) and CCND1 (10%, amplification). Tumors harboring these alterations may be amenable to cyclin-dependent kinase inhibitors such as palbociclib or LEE011. Chromatin regulatory genes were altered in 76% of tumors in the bladder TCGA. Although the biological ramifications of such alterations have yet to be elucidated, evidence for the utility of histone deacetylase inhibitors in UC already exist: in one phase I trial of vorinostat in advanced solid tumor patients, 2 metastatic UC patients experienced responses lasting 6 and 7 months, respectively; in a second trial, 1 of 7 metastatic UC patients exhibited SD for 10 months.[64,65] A trial of the histone deacetylase inhibitor mocetinostat in advanced UC patients with CREBBP or EP300 alterations is ongoing.

SUMMARY

Metastatic UC is a lethal disease, and platinum-based chemotherapy remains the optimum first-line therapy. Although phase I and II trials of targeted agents have not displayed a significant improvement in survival or response when compared with cytotoxic therapy, a common theme has been the lack of genetic preselection of patients enrolled onto these studies. Several studies in other cancer types have found that those patients whose tumors harbor a specific genetic target are most likely to respond to small molecule inhibitor treatments, with the requirement that the molecular target of these inhibitors is well defined. With the advent of next-generation sequencing technologies, both deep coverage exon capture sequencing and unbiased exome or genome sequencing, new trials of targeted agents are underway that incorporate the presence of specific genetic aberrations into enrollment criteria. Additionally, basket studies, in which a drug is tested across tumor types and enrollment is based principally on the presence of specific genetic alterations within a gene or genes, represent a unique trial design to rapidly screen the efficacy of targeted agents and define the predictive capacity of the same aberration in different tumors. Finally, it should be noted that although novel sequencing technologies have unearthed several somatic alterations in UC, a better understanding of the functional consequences, relevance to tumorigenesis, and drug sensitivity of many of these alterations (ie, identifying the true drivers of oncogenesis) are still required and will hopefully inform clinical trials of targeted therapies for this disease in the future.

REFERENCES

1. Siegel R, Ma J, Zou Z, et al. Cancer statistics, 2014. CA Cancer J Clin 2014;64(1):9–29.

2. von der Maase H, Sengelov L, Roberts JT, et al. Long-term survival results of a randomized trial comparing gemcitabine plus cisplatin, with methotrexate, vinblastine, doxorubicin, plus cisplatin in patients with bladder cancer. J Clin Oncol 2005;23(21):4602–8.

3. Bellmunt J, von der Maase H, Mead GM, et al. Randomized phase III study comparing paclitaxel/cisplatin/gemcitabine and gemcitabine/cisplatin in patients with locally advanced or metastatic urothelial cancer without prior systemic therapy: EORTC Intergroup Study 30987. J Clin Oncol 2012;30(10):1107–13.

4. Sternberg CN, de Mulder PH, Schornagel JH, et al, European Organization for Research and Treatment of Cancer Genitourinary Tract Cancer Cooperative Group. Randomized phase III trial of high-dose-intensity methotrexate, vinblastine, doxorubicin, and cisplatin (MVAC) chemotherapy and recombinant human granulocyte colony-stimulating factor versus classic MVAC in advanced urothelial tract tumors: European Organization for Research and Treatment of Cancer Protocol no. 30924. J Clin Oncol 2001;19(10):2638–46.

5. Dovedi SJ, Davies BR. Emerging targeted therapies for bladder cancer: a disease waiting for a drug. Cancer Metastasis Rev 2009;28(3–4):355–67.

6. Zhang ZT, Pak J, Huang HY, et al. Role of Ha-ras activation in superficial papillary pathway of urothelial tumor formation. Oncogene 2001;20(16):1973–80.

7. Bakkar AA, Wallerand H, Radvanyi F, et al. FGFR3 and TP53 gene mutations define two distinct pathways in urothelial cell carcinoma of the bladder. Cancer Res 2003;63(23):8108–12.

8. Cancer Genome Atlas Research Network. Comprehensive molecular characterization of urothelial bladder carcinoma. Nature 2014;507(7492):315–22.

9. Iyer G, Al-Ahmadie H, Schultz N, et al. Prevalence and co-occurrence of actionable genomic alterations in high-grade bladder cancer. J Clin Oncol 2013;31(25):3133–40.

10. Bellmunt J, Hussain M, Dinney CP. Novel approaches with targeted therapies in bladder cancer. Therapy of bladder cancer by blockade of the epidermal growth factor receptor family. Crit Rev Oncol Hematol 2003;46(Suppl):S85–104.

11. Nutt JE, Lazarowicz HP, Mellon JK, et al. Gefitinib ('Iressa', ZD1839) inhibits the growth response of bladder tumour cell lines to epidermal growth factor and induces TIMP2. Br J Cancer 2004;90(8):1679–85.

12. Petrylak DP, Tangen CM, Van Veldhuizen PJ Jr, et al. Results of the Southwest Oncology Group phase II evaluation (study S0031) of ZD1839 for advanced transitional cell carcinoma of the urothelium. BJU Int 2010;105(3):317–21.

13. Philips GK, Halabi S, Sanford BL, et al. A phase II trial of cisplatin (C), gemcitabine (G) and gefitinib for advanced urothelial tract carcinoma: results of Cancer and Leukemia Group B (CALGB) 90102. Ann Oncol 2009;20(6):1074–9.

14. Pruthi RS, Nielsen M, Heathcote S, et al. A phase II trial of neoadjuvant erlotinib in patients with muscle-invasive bladder cancer undergoing radical cystectomy: clinical and pathological results. BJU Int 2010;106(3):349–54.

15. Wulfing C, Machiels JP, Richel DJ, et al. A single-arm, multicenter, open-label phase 2 study of lapatinib as the second-line treatment of patients with locally advanced or metastatic transitional cell carcinoma. Cancer 2009;115(13):2881–90.

16. Vermorken JB, Mesia R, Rivera F, et al. Platinum-based chemotherapy plus cetuximab in head and neck cancer. N Engl J Med 2008;359(11):1116–27.

17. Van Cutsem E, Kohne CH, Hitre E, et al. Cetuximab and chemotherapy as initial treatment for metastatic colorectal cancer. N Engl J Med 2009;360(14):1408–17.

18. Van Cutsem E, Kohne CH, Lang I, et al. Cetuximab plus irinotecan, fluorouracil, and leucovorin as first-line treatment for metastatic colorectal cancer: updated analysis of overall survival according to tumor KRAS and BRAF mutation status. J Clin Oncol 2011;29(15):2011–9.

19. Wong YN, Litwin S, Vaughn D, et al. Phase II trial of cetuximab with or without paclitaxel in patients with advanced urothelial tract carcinoma. J Clin Oncol 2012;30(28):3545–51.

20. Hussain M, Daignault S, Agarwal N, et al. A randomized phase 2 trial of gemcitabine/cisplatin with or without cetuximab in patients with advanced urothelial carcinoma. Cancer 2014;120(17):2684–93.

21. Simonetti S, Russo R, Ciancia G, et al. Role of polysomy 17 in transitional cell carcinoma of the bladder: immunohistochemical study of HER2/neu expression and fish analysis of c-erbB-2 gene and chromosome 17. Int J Surg Pathol 2009;17(3):198–205.

22. Inoue T, Sato K, Tsuchiya N, et al. Numeric aberrations of HER-2 and chromosome 17 detected by fluorescence in situ hybridization in urine-exfoliated cells from patients with urothelial carcinoma. Urology 2004;64(3):617–21.

23. Schneider SA, Sukov WR, Frank I, et al. Outcome of patients with micropapillary urothelial carcinoma following radical cystectomy: ERBB2 (HER2)

amplification identifies patients with poor outcome. Mod Pathol 2014;27(5):758–64.

24. Hussain MH, MacVicar GR, Petrylak DP, et al. Trastuzumab, paclitaxel, carboplatin, and gemcitabine in advanced human epidermal growth factor receptor-2/neu-positive urothelial carcinoma: results of a multicenter phase II National Cancer Institute trial. J Clin Oncol 2007;25(16):2218–24.

25. Rabindran SK, Discafani CM, Rosfjord EC, et al. Antitumor activity of HKI-272, an orally active, irreversible inhibitor of the HER-2 tyrosine kinase. Cancer Res 2004;64(11):3958–65.

26. Saura C, Garcia-Saenz JA, Xu B, et al. Safety and efficacy of neratinib in combination with capecitabine in patients with metastatic human epidermal growth factor receptor 2-positive breast cancer. J Clin Oncol 2014;32(32):3626–33.

27. Katoh M, Nakagama H. FGF receptors: cancer biology and therapeutics. Med Res Rev 2014; 34(2):280–300.

28. Milowsky MI, Dittrich C, Duran I, et al. Phase 2 trial of dovitinib in patients with progressive FGFR3-mutated or FGFR3 wild-type advanced urothelial carcinoma. Eur J Cancer 2014;50(18):3145–52.

29. Sequist LV. Phase I study of BGJ398, a selective pan-FGFR inhibitor in genetically preselected advanced solid tumors. Proceedings of the 105th Annual Meeting of the American Association for Cancer Research. San Diego (CA); Philadelphia, April 5–9, 2014. AACR; 2014. Abstract CT326, 2014.

30. Coultas L, Chawengsaksophak K, Rossant J. Endothelial cells and VEGF in vascular development. Nature 2005;438(7070):937–45.

31. Kopparapu PK, Boorjian SA, Robinson BD, et al. Expression of VEGF and its receptors VEGFR1/VEGFR2 is associated with invasiveness of bladder cancer. Anticancer Res 2013;33(6):2381–90.

32. Inoue K, Slaton JW, Kim SJ, et al. Interleukin 8 expression regulates tumorigenicity and metastasis in human bladder cancer. Cancer Res 2000;60(8): 2290–9.

33. Allen LE, Maher PA. Expression of basic fibroblast growth factor and its receptor in an invasive bladder carcinoma cell line. J Cell Physiol 1993;155(2):368–75.

34. Huang YJ, Qi WX, He AN, et al. Prognostic value of tissue vascular endothelial growth factor expression in bladder cancer: a meta-analysis. Asian Pac J Cancer Prev 2013;14(2):645–9.

35. Bochner BH, Cote RJ, Weidner N, et al. Angiogenesis in bladder cancer: relationship between microvessel density and tumor prognosis. J Natl Cancer Inst 1995;87(21):1603–12.

36. Inoue K, Slaton JW, Karashima T, et al. The prognostic value of angiogenesis factor expression for predicting recurrence and metastasis of bladder cancer after neoadjuvant chemotherapy and radical cystectomy. Clin Cancer Res 2000;6(12):4866–73.

37. Sonpavde G, Jian W, Liu H, et al. Sunitinib malate is active against human urothelial carcinoma and enhances the activity of cisplatin in a preclinical model. Urol Oncol 2009;27(4):391–9.

38. Gallagher DJ, Milowsky MI, Gerst SR, et al. Phase II study of sunitinib in patients with metastatic urothelial cancer. J Clin Oncol 2010;28(8):1373–9.

39. Galsky MD, Hahn NM, Powles T, et al. Gemcitabine, Cisplatin, and sunitinib for metastatic urothelial carcinoma and as preoperative therapy for muscle-invasive bladder cancer. Clin Genitourin Cancer 2013;11(2):175–81.

40. Bellmunt J, Gonzalez-Larriba JL, Prior C, et al. Phase II study of sunitinib as first-line treatment of urothelial cancer patients ineligible to receive cisplatin-based chemotherapy: baseline interleukin-8 and tumor contrast enhancement as potential predictive factors of activity. Ann Oncol 2011;22(12):2646–53.

41. Sridhar SS, Winquist E, Eisen A, et al. A phase II trial of sorafenib in first-line metastatic urothelial cancer: a study of the PMH Phase II Consortium. Invest New Drugs 2011;29(5):1045–9.

42. Dreicer R, Li H, Stein M, et al. Phase 2 trial of sorafenib in patients with advanced urothelial cancer: a trial of the Eastern Cooperative Oncology Group. Cancer 2009;115(18):4090–5.

43. Krege S, Rexer H, vom Dorp F, et al. Prospective randomized double-blind multicentre phase II study comparing gemcitabine and cisplatin plus sorafenib chemotherapy with gemcitabine and cisplatin plus placebo in locally advanced and/or metastasized urothelial cancer: SUSE (AUO-AB 31/05). BJU Int 2014;113(3):429–36.

44. Hamberg P, Verweij J, Sleijfer S. (Pre-)clinical pharmacology and activity of pazopanib, a novel multikinase angiogenesis inhibitor. Oncologist 2010;15(6):539–47.

45. Necchi A, Mariani L, Zaffaroni N, et al. Pazopanib in advanced and platinum-resistant urothelial cancer: an open-label, single group, phase 2 trial. Lancet Oncol 2012;13(8):810–6.

46. Choueiri TK, Ross RW, Jacobus S, et al. Double-blind, randomized trial of docetaxel plus vandetanib versus docetaxel plus placebo in platinum-pretreated metastatic urothelial cancer. J Clin Oncol 2012;30(5):507–12.

47. Bellmunt J, Choueiri TK, Fougeray R, et al. Prognostic factors in patients with advanced transitional cell carcinoma of the urothelial tract experiencing treatment failure with platinum-containing regimens. J Clin Oncol 2010;28(11):1850–5.

48. Escudier B, Pluzanska A, Koralewski P, et al. Bevacizumab plus interferon alfa-2a for treatment of metastatic renal cell carcinoma: a randomised, double-blind phase III trial. Lancet 2007;370(9605): 2103–11.

49. Friedman HS, Prados MD, Wen PY, et al. Bevacizumab alone and in combination with irinotecan in

recurrent glioblastoma. J Clin Oncol 2009;27(28): 4733–40.

50. Hurwitz H, Fehrenbacher L, Novotny W, et al. Bevacizumab plus irinotecan, fluorouracil, and leucovorin for metastatic colorectal cancer. N Engl J Med 2004; 350(23):2335–42.

51. Kreisl TN, Kim L, Moore K, et al. Phase II trial of single-agent bevacizumab followed by bevacizumab plus irinotecan at tumor progression in recurrent glioblastoma. J Clin Oncol 2009;27(5): 740–5.

52. Rini BI, Halabi S, Rosenberg JE, et al. Bevacizumab plus interferon alfa compared with interferon alfa monotherapy in patients with metastatic renal cell carcinoma: CALGB 90206. J Clin Oncol 2008; 26(33):5422–8.

53. Sandler A, Gray R, Perry MC, et al. Paclitaxel-carboplatin alone or with bevacizumab for non-small-cell lung cancer. N Engl J Med 2006;355(24):2542–50.

54. Hahn NM, Stadler WM, Zon RT, et al. Phase II trial of cisplatin, gemcitabine, and bevacizumab as first-line therapy for metastatic urothelial carcinoma: Hoosier Oncology Group GU 04–75. J Clin Oncol 2011;29(12):1525–30.

55. Balar AV, Apolo AB, Ostrovnaya I, et al. Phase II study of gemcitabine, carboplatin, and bevacizumab in patients with advanced unresectable or metastatic urothelial cancer. J Clin Oncol 2013;31(6): 724–30.

56. Laplante M, Sabatini DM. mTOR signaling in growth control and disease. Cell 2012;149(2):274–93.

57. Motzer RJ, Escudier B, Oudard S, et al. Efficacy of everolimus in advanced renal cell carcinoma: a double-blind, randomised, placebo-controlled phase III trial. Lancet 2008;372(9637):449–56.

58. Yao JC, Shah MH, Ito T, et al, T.T.S.G. Rad001 in Advanced Neuroendocrine Tumors. Everolimus for advanced pancreatic neuroendocrine tumors. N Engl J Med 2011;364(6):514–23.

59. Baselga J, Campone M, Piccart M, et al. Everolimus in postmenopausal hormone-receptor-positive advanced breast cancer. N Engl J Med 2012;366(6): 520–9.

60. Mansure JJ, Nassim R, Chevalier S, et al. Inhibition of mammalian target of rapamycin as a therapeutic strategy in the management of bladder cancer. Cancer Biol Ther 2009;8(24):2339–47.

61. Seront E, Rottey S, Sautois B, et al. Phase II study of everolimus in patients with locally advanced or metastatic transitional cell carcinoma of the urothelial tract: clinical activity, molecular response, and biomarkers. Ann Oncol 2012;23(10):2663–70.

62. Milowsky MI, Iyer G, Regazzi AM, et al. Phase II study of everolimus in metastatic urothelial cancer. BJU Int 2013;112(4):462–70.

63. Iyer G, Hanrahan AJ, Milowsky MI, et al. Genome sequencing identifies a basis for everolimus sensitivity. Science 2012;338(6104):221.

64. Kelly WK, Richon VM, O'Connor O, et al. Phase I clinical trial of histone deacetylase inhibitor: suberoylanilide hydroxamic acid administered intravenously. Clin Cancer Res 2003;9(10 Pt 1):3578–88.

65. Kelly WK, O'Connor OA, Krug LM, et al. Phase I study of an oral histone deacetylase inhibitor, suberoylanilide hydroxamic acid, in patients with advanced cancer. J Clin Oncol 2005;23(17):3923–31.

Index

Note: Page numbers of article titles are in **boldface** type.

Urol Clin N Am 42 (2015) 263–268
http://dx.doi.org/10.1016/S0094-0143(15)00023-3
0094-0143/15/$ – see front matter © 2015 Elsevier Inc. All rights reserved.

Printed and bound by CPI Group (UK) Ltd, Croydon, CR0 4YY

03/10/2024

01040375-0008